DIRECT VERSUS INDIRECT REALISM

DIRECT VERSUS INDIRECT REALISM

A Neurophilosophical Debate on Consciousness

Edited by

JOHN SMYTHIES
The Center for Brain and Cognition,
University of California San Diego, La Jolla, CA, United States

ROBERT FRENCH
Adjunct Instructor, Philosophy,
Oakland Community College,
Waterford Township, MI, United States

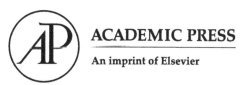

ACADEMIC PRESS

An imprint of Elsevier

Academic Press is an imprint of Elsevier
125 London Wall, London EC2Y 5AS, United Kingdom
525 B Street, Suite 1800, San Diego, CA 92101-4495, United States
50 Hampshire Street, 5th Floor, Cambridge, MA 02139, United States
The Boulevard, Langford Lane, Kidlington, Oxford OX5 1GB, United Kingdom

Library of Congress Cataloging-in-Publication Data
A catalog record for this book is available from the Library of Congress

British Library Cataloguing-in-Publication Data
A catalogue record for this book is available from the British Library

ISBN: 978-0-12-812141-2

For information on all Academic Press publications visit our website at
https://www.elsevier.com/books-and-journals

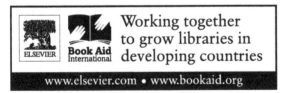

Working together
to grow libraries in
developing countries

www.elsevier.com • www.bookaid.org

Publisher: Niki Levy
Acquisition Editor: Joslyn Paguio
Editorial Project Manager: Gabriela Capille
Production Project Manager: Anusha Sambamoorthy
Cover Designer: Miles Hitchen

Typeset by TNQ Books and Journals

CONTENTS

LIST OF CONTRIBUTORS

Fred Adams
Linguistics & Cognitive Science and Philosophy, University of Delaware, Newark, DE, United States

Murray Clarke
Philosophy, Concordia University, Montreal, Canada

William Fish
Philosophy Department, Massey University, Palmerston North, New Zealand

Robert French
Adjunct Instructor, Philosophy, Oakland Community College, Waterford Township, MI, United States

Gary Fuller
Philosophy, Central Michigan University, Mt. Pleasant, MI, United States

Michael Huemer
Department of Philosophy, University of Colorado, Boulder, CO, United States

Ernest W. Kent
Formerly: Chief Scientist, Intelligent Systems Division, The National Institute of Standards and Technology, Gaithersburg, MD, United States; Formerly: Director of Research in Information Technology for N. America, Phillips, N.V., Briarcliff Manor, NY, United States; Formerly: Associate Professor of Physiological Psychology and Psychopharmacology, The University of Illinois at Chicago, Chicago, IL, United States

Pierre Le Morvan
Department of Philosophy, Religion, and Classical Studies, The College of New Jersey, Ewing, NJ, United States

Steven Lehar
Independent Researcher, Manchester, MA, United States

David McGraw
Adjunct Professor, Philosophy, Wayne County Community College, Detroit, MI, United States

Eva Schmidt
Philosophy Department, University of Zürich (UZH), Zürich, Switzerland

John Smythies
The Center for Brain and Cognition, University of California San Diego, La Jolla, CA, United States

ACKNOWLEDGMENTS

For the cover image we would like to acknowledge Robin Siegel, inspired by Joan Miró, for creating the image, to Stephanie Smythies for her help over style, and to Larry Edelstein for his help relating to matters of copyright.

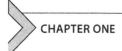

CHAPTER ONE

Introduction

John Smythies[1], Robert French[2]
[1]The Center for Brain and Cognition, University of California San Diego, La Jolla, CA, United States;
[2]Adjunct Instructor, Philosophy, Oakland Community College, Waterford Township, MI, United States

We believe that the current state of affairs in the philosophy of perception is not entirely healthy. On the one hand, the dominant position among philosophers working in the philosophy of perception is "direct realism"—the claim that the immediate objects of perception are distal physical objects. Grounds here include (1) the claim that the position fits in better with the naturalistic metaphysics of physical science, there being no need to posit a separate phenomenal realm apart from the physical; (2) that it is in better accord with common sense and the ordinary language of perception; e.g., we ordinarily speak of perceiving physical objects not phenomenal ones; and (3) that it is epistemically more straightforward, there being no inference involved with visual perception, for example, we just open our eyes and are immediately aware of distant objects. In fact this position has become so dominant in the current literature in the philosophy of mind that other positions are typically either completely ignored or just summarily dismissed without even bothering to say why.

In contrast the situation is very different among people actually working in the neurosciences. There it is felt that there is overwhelming evidence from the brain sciences that conscious experiences consist of reconstructions from information encoded in neural states and is hence indirect.

For example,

- It has been well established by numerous experiments that we see, not what is actually "out there" but what the brain computes is most probably "out there."
- In vision, processings of color, shape, and motion of visual stimuli are carried out not only in quite different locations in the visual brain but also at different speeds, color being the fastest followed by shape and motion. Somehow at the highest level all these separate computations are amalgamated into the unified visual object that we see.
- Neuroplasticity experiments have shown that visual neurons (stimulation of which results in a conscious visual experience) can be changed

Direct versus Indirect Realism
ISBN 978-0-12-812141-2
https://doi.org/10.1016/B978-0-12-812141-2.00001-5

by epigenetic manipulations into functioning auditory neurons, stimulation of which results in a conscious auditory experience. Furthermore, it has been shown that stimulation by a flickering light of a visual cortical neuron via its usual input from the retina from the connected open eye results in one type of visual experience (geometrical patterns), whereas uniocular stimulation of the same neuron by the corticocortical route results in a quite different conscious visual experience ("oily swirls").

• It has been shown that a prominent mechanism used by the visual brain is information compression. In this process an incoming visual picture, relayed from the retina to the cortex, is divided into successive frames. The first frame is imprinted on the lower visual cortex (V1) and then transmitted to the higher visual cortex. Then the second frame is imprinted on top of the first frame and information common to both frames is deleted and only the differences between the two frames are transmitted to the higher visual cortex. This process repeats for all successive frames. This mechanism results in considerable savings of computational resources. It also entails that different areas of the visual field have different origins. At the focus of attention what is seen is based on information provided directly from the retina. Whereas in the unattended-to background, the picture is built up from memories stored in the higher visual cortex.

These facts are difficult to account for in any direct realist theory of vision.

It is our strong opinion that in the interest of seeking truth, there is a lot to be said for having people with strongly opposing positions, such as in this case, not just talk among themselves but to interact with people from the other side. Thus we have set up this book in the format of a debate, whereby people on each side are given the opportunity to state an initial position. People on the other side are then given the opportunity to present a statement of rebuttal. Finally the original side is given the opportunity to respond to the rebuttals. We have tried hard to make the debate a fair debate and to have strong proponents of each side be represented. We have also strived to cover a diversity of aspects of both positions while avoiding duplication of content. We allow readers to judge who has come up with the stronger positions.

We decided to keep participation in the debate portion of the anthology voluntary. Thus, the fact that there is no reply by original authors in some cases on both sides of the debate should not be taken as evidence of agreement with the criticisms. Also, there are obvious disagreements among the authors within both the direct and indirect realists' camps, but we do not address these.

PART ONE

Papers Defending Indirect Realism

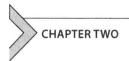

CHAPTER TWO

The Metaphysical Foundations of Contemporary Neuroscience: A House Built on Sand

John Smythies
The Center for Brain and Cognition, University of California San Diego, La Jolla, CA, United States

1. INTRODUCTION

By "metaphysics" I mean the series of assumptions, often unconscious and taken for granted, made by the scientist that underlie her arguments when she constructs her hypotheses in neuroscience related in particular to the problem of consciousness.

This paper reviews such assumptions in three different but interconnected areas:

- The underlying cosmological theory—whether Newtonian or special relativity (SR). This involves the treatment of space, time, and matter by the theory.
- The theory of perception used—direct realism or the representative theory—whether formally or smuggled in. A subset of this section is the treatment of the concept of the body image. This involves the proposed relationship between phenomenal objects and external physical objects.
- The account the hypothesis gives of the ontological relation between certain brain events called the neural correlates of consciousness (NCCs) and the related phenomenal events that we experience in consciousness (i.e., our sensations, images, feelings, and thoughts). The point at issue is whether the relation between them is one of identity—as in the Identity theory (IT)—or one of causality.

2. THE COSMOLOGICAL THEORY

The world is described by Newtonian theory as a collection of 3D objects extended in a 3D space. They exist in a separate time that flows independently. Their movement in space during time is determined by Newton's laws of motion—in particular his law of gravity that describes

Direct versus Indirect Realism
ISBN 978-0-12-812141-2
https://doi.org/10.1016/B978-0-12-812141-2.00002-7

gravity is an attractive force between objects. SR, however, unites time and space into a 4D space-time. Objects cease to be 3D spatial entities that exist in a separate ID time and become stationary 4D world lines that extend from the beginning to the end of the Universe. The earth is not a 3D body that circles round the sun, but a 4D hyperhelix that is wound in a stationary spiral form about the world lines of the 4D sun. The apparent movement of objects is an illusion generated by the movement of the Observer in space-time along the time dimension. This involves the existence of two types of time (1) the fourth spacelike dimension of space-time and (2) real-time t2 in which the Observer moves. Gravity as a force is abolished, to be replaced by pure geometry. The following is a list of comments by leading physicists, philosophers, and neuroscientists on this subject:

- Louis de Broglie (1959):

  Each observer, as his time passes, discovers, so to speak, new slices of space-time which appear to him as successive aspects of the material world, though in reality the ensemble of events constituting space-time exist prior to his knowledge of them… the aggregate of past, present and future phenomena are in some sense given a priori.

- Stannard (1987):

  Physics itself recognizes no special moment called 'now'—the moment that acts as the focus of 'becoming' and divides the 'past' from the 'future'. In four-dimensional space-time nothing changes, there is no flow of time, everything simply is… It is only in consciousness that we come across the particular time known as 'now'… It is only in the context of mental time that it makes sense to say that all of physical space-time is. One might even go so far as to say that it is unfortunate that such dissimilar entities as physical time and mental time should carry the same name!

- Lord Brain (1963):

  Moreover when we describe what happens in the nervous system when we are concerned with the movement of electrical impulses in space (i.e. along neurons), and though we use physical time to describe these movements, we can never abstract from such an account time as we experience it psychologically.

- Penrose (1994) says that in SR

  …particles do not even move, being represented by 'static' curves drawn in space-time. Thus what we perceive as moving 3D objects are really successive cross-sections of immobile 4D objects past which our field of observation is sweeping.

- Quine (1982): "A drastic departure from English is required in the matter of time. The view to adopt is the Minkowskian one, which sees time as a fourth dimension on a par with the three dimensions of space."

- Lloyd (1978): "For the Quinean, what differences we see between past, present and future pertain to our limited mode of access to reality."
- Heller (1984): "I propose that a physical object is not an enduring hunk of matter but an enduring spatio-temporal hunk of matter."
- Eddington (1920): "Events do not happen: they are just there, and we come across them... [as]... the observer on his voyage of exploration."
- Weyl (1949): "The objective world simply *is*, it does not *happen*. Only to the gaze of my consciousness crawling upward along the life-line [world line] of my body does a section of this world come to life as a fleeting image."
- Werth (1978) draws attention to the fact that this is the case for somatic sensation as well as to vision: he says,

  Our apparent body ['body image' is the neurological name for this] at each instant is simply a 'slice' of our four-dimensional body. That is the experiencing subject sequentially 'intersects' his four-dimensional body and 'projects' the sequence of three-dimensional intersections upon the 'screen' of his consciousness: his body appears to him as being ever changing though in physical reality it is a static and immutable four-dimensional object.

- Lastly Broad (1953) presents the logic that underlies this argument in his usual meticulous fashion:
- "...if we assume one additional spatial dimension beside the three we can observe, and if we suppose that our field of observation at any one moment is confined to the content of a {3,4}-fold which moves uniformly at right angles to itself along a straight line in the {3,4}-fold, then there is no need to assume *any other* motion in the universe. This *one uniform rectilinear* motion of *the observer's field of observation*, together with the *purely geometrical properties* of the *stationary* material *threads* in the four-fold, will account for all the various observed motions (various in both magnitude and direction) of the material *particles* which are the appearances of these threads in the successive fields of observation."

However, we are still faced with the problem of the nature of this "observer" invoked by several of these statements (e.g., De Broglie, Lloyd, and Broad). This does not refer as to the physical body of the scientist, which is composed (like all physical objects) of its stationary world lines extended on space–time, but to a Self or Observer that can move in time in the way described. In the block universe, consciousness and the Self are located at the experienced moving "now" of time. As Alexander (1975) says "...the present being a moment of physical Time fixed by relation to an observing mind." Thus the observer in a block universe with a shifting "now" of time must be some entity in addition to the physical body.

In spite of the fact that SR has been known for a century to be correct and Newtonian theory only an approximation, all the theories of biology, evolution, and neuroscience today still remain resolutely rooted in the Newtonian system. For example, evolutionary theory today describes 3D organisms competing in a 3D space in a separate time and changing their structures dynamically as they do so. Whereas all these dynamic changes are described in SR as features of the static 4D sculpture of the world lines of these organisms. If all the experts quoted earlier are correct, these organisms only appear to be moving because they are being observed by the Observer on its time travel along their common time dimension. If so, radical changes are needed in our idea of "evolution." Organisms do not evolve in a block universe—rather the observer sees successive cross sections of the organism's 4D physical structure that is simply more complex the further up the time dimension the observer travels. This realization also requires radical changes in our ideas of what brain "events" actually consist of in a Minkowskian block universe. Brain "events" are not composed of moving 3D atoms but of successive 3D cross sections of the static 4D world lines of these atoms. SR replaces 3D "movement" by weaving patterns of complex 4D geometry, or sculpture, at the neural as well as the cosmic scale. However, this does not require any changes in practical day-to-day experimental neuroscience for which Newtonian terminology is quite sufficient. The need to consider the SR picture only comes in effect when deeper questions as to the nature of reality are being asked.

3. TWO COMPETING THEORIES OF PERCEPTION

Contemporary neuroscience presents a strange and confused picture in the field of perception. There are essentially two theories of perception competing today. The first is naïve realism (NR). This is the theory of "common sense," held by all ordinary people and many philosophers. It says that, in perception, we are directly acquainted with external physical objects. When I open my eyes, the large white object that springs into my visual field simply is my car, or at least its surface. All that my brain does is to allow this to happen in some way explainable by some philosophers to their own satisfaction by complex Wittgensteinian arguments. Unfortunately, there is now a mountain of evidence from neuroscience itself that this is quite wrong and that the rival Representative Theory is right.

In vision, we do not experience the world as it actually is, but as the brain computes it most probably to be (Vernon, 1962; Gregory, 1981;

Ramachandran and Blakeslee, 1998; Smythies and Ramachandran, 1998; Kleiser et al., 2004; Kovács et al., 1996; Yarrow et al., 2001). As Crick (1994) put it "What you see is not what is really there; it is what your brain believes is there." Visual sensations are not composed of external objects, as the Direct Realist theory suggests, but are constructed by the representative mechanisms of perception. In vision, color, shape, and movement are processed by separate mechanisms located in different parts of the brain. These operate at different speeds, so that we actually see the color of an object before its shape, and its shape before is motion (Zeki, 2015). The time differences are small—40 ms in each case—so that we do not notice it in ordinary vision, just as we do not notice the blind spot in our visual field, but Zeki by clever experiments has shown that they exist. It is interesting that the same system holds in modern digital TV. TV designers have discovered that the best way to transmit and process the TV signal is to compute color, form, and motion separately (Smythies and Doreye, 2016). They did not discover this by finding out how the visual brain works and copying that but by doing experiments of their own.

The same logic applies to somatic sensation. Almost everyone believes today that we experience our physical bodies directly in consciousness. We wake up feeling ensconced in our bodies "like a pilot in his vessel" as Descartes put it—just "my oh-so-familiar body" that is with us all day long, parts of which we can move at will. However, this is a mistake. Neurological investigations of the complex phenomena of "phantom" limbs show that all bodily sensations—including "phantom" limbs—cannot be identical with events in the physical body but only with events in the parietal cortex (Schilder, 1950; Smythies, 1953; Ramachandran and Blakeslee, 1998). As the Viennese neurologist Paul Schilder (1950) said "…the empirical method leads immediately to a deep insight that even our own body is beyond our immediate reach, that even our own body justifies Prospero's words" "We are such stuff as dreams are made on, and our little life is rounded with a sleep".

Wolfgang Köhler, a founder of Gestalt psychology, made this very clear (1947):

Rather, I learned that physical objects influence a particularly interesting physical system, my organism, and that my objective experience results when, as a consequence, certain complicated processes have happened in that system. Obviously, I realized, I cannot identify the final products, the things and events of that experience, with the physical objects from which the influences came… My body [somatic sensory field or body image] is the outcome of certain processes in my physical organism, processes which start in the eyes, muscles, skin and so forth, exactly as the chair before me is the final product of other processes in the same physical organism. If the chair is seen 'before me', the 'me' of this phrase means my body as an experience, of course, not my organism as an object in the physical world.

Searle (1992) is one of the very rare philosophers to understand this:

The brain creates a body image, and pains, like all bodily sensations, are parts of the body image. The pain-in-the-foot is literally in the physical space of the brain.

The neurologist Jason Brown (1991) put it well

Space itself is an object: volumetric, egocentric, and part of the mind of the observer… Mind is positioned in a space of its own making… We wonder about the limits of the universe but never ask what is beyond the space of a dream.

This point can be made by asking someone to point to where, in the world they experience, their brain is located. They will point at once to the head that they experience. This is a mistake—how can the brain be in the experienced head when the experienced head is in the brain?

4. THE IDENTITY THEORY AND THE STATUS OF PHENOMENAL SPACE

The IT states that the NCCs are identical with particular electro-chemical activities in certain nerve nets in the brain. Most neuroscientists hold tenaciously to this hypothesis. However, there are serious difficulties with it. The events in consciousness that we experience consist of a number of phenomenal events—our sensations, images, thoughts, and feelings. Psychologists can examine these by introspection and determine their properties. In vision we can observe that phenomenal objects have the properties of particular color(s), geometrical form and geometrical relation, and motion. As Quinton (1962) says: "My visual sense–data [sensations] are extended spatial entities, occupying positions and spatially interrelated to other things in the space of my momentary visual field… My after–image is plainly a spatial thing, it occupies at any one moment a definite position in my visual field…" Psychologists (such as Gregory, 1981; Vernon, 1962; Ramachandran and Blakeslee, 1998; Smythies and Ramachandran, 1998; Smythies, 1959a,b, 1960) have conducted extensive experiments into such phenomena as a wide range of the effects of brain injuries on perception, the filling-in of scotomata, constancy effects, the stroboscopic phenomena, number forms, hallucinations of various kinds, synesthesiae, afterimages, eidetic images, and many more. These experiments give us important information about the perceptual process that could not have been obtained by neurophysiological or brain imaging techniques—for example, "This afterimage is red, round and in the center of my visual field" and "These three afterimages are arranged in the form of a triangle."

Leibniz's law of the Identity of Indiscernibles states, "For two entities to be identical they must have all properties in common." Plainly electrochemical activity in a distributed nerve net in the brain has few, if any, properties in common with the phenomenal object it gives rise to. The two entities or activities can be *correlated*, but they cannot be *identical*. In particular this may involve the fact that the two may lie in different space systems. Bertrand Russell (1948) puts this clearly:

> The objects of perception which I take to be 'external' to me, such as coloured surfaces that I see, are only 'external' in my private space... When on a common-sense basis, people talk of the gulf between mind and matter, what they really have in mind is the gulf between a tactual percept, and a 'thought'—e.g. a memory, a pleasure, or a volition. But this, as we have seen, is a division within the mental world; the percept is as mental as the 'thought'.

Furthermore, the relationship of identity is transitive and operates in both directions. If *a* is identical to *b* then *b* is identical to *a*. Neuroscientists may have got used to the idea that NCCs may be identical to phenomenal events. When they look at the mass of pink jelly that is a brain they can say to themselves "Somewhere in there are sensations and thoughts." However, they are not used to the idea that phenomenal events are identical to NCCs. When they examine one of their own visual sensations they do not think "This entity before me out there now is literally constructed of my neurons" as their own hypothesis claims it is.

The theoretical physicist Andrei Linde (1990) has suggested that the world consists of three different fundamental constituents—[physical] space-time, matter, and consciousness, each with their own degrees of freedom. The neuroscientist Hartwig Kuhlenbeck (1958) says that "...physical events and mental events occur in different space-time systems which have no dimensions in common."

Common sense believes that there is only one space (space-time) in the world and that phenomenal space is merely the way physical space appears to us. In his recent book Stephen Hawking (2001) says: "It is a matter of common experience that we live in a three-dimensional space. That is to say, we can represent the position of a point in space by three numbers, for example, latitude, longitude, and height above sea level." We can certainly do this with physical space. However, we do not experience physical space or its contents. What we experience is phenomenal space, and the relationship between physical space and phenomenal space is certainly not a "matter of common experience" but is the subject of intense debate that has raised the possibility that phenomenal space and physical space are ontologically and geometrically different spaces (Broad, 1923; Price, 1953). The private space we inhabit during a dream undeniably has geometrical properties. For further developments of this theme see Smythies (1994a,b, 2009, 2013, 2014), French (1987), and see the astrophysicist Bernard Carr (2008) for an extensive review from the point of view of cosmology.

ACKNOWLEDGMENTS

Portions of this review are taken from a previous review in the Italian cultural publication "Il Cannochiale" issue 1/2016.

REFERENCES

Alexander, S., 1975. Time and space. In: Shearer, C.M. (Ed.), The Human Experience of Time. New York University Press, New York.
Brain, L., 1963. Some reflections on brain and mind. Brain 86, 381–402.
Broad, C.D., 1923. Scientific Thought. Routledge & Kegan Paul, London.
Broad, C.D., 1953. Religion, Philosophy and Psychical Research. Routledge & Kegan Paul, London.
Brown, J.W., 1991. Self and Process. Springer-Verlag, New York.
Carr, B., 2008. Worlds apart? Proc. Soc. Psych. Res. 59, 1–96.
Crick, F., 1994. The Astonishing Hypothesis. Scribner, New York.
de Broglie, L., 1959. A general survey of the scientific work of Albert Einstein. In: Schlipp, P.A. (Ed.), Albert Einstein Philosopher-Scientist. Harper & Row, New York, pp. 107–128.
Eddington, A., 1920, Space, Time, and Gravitation: An Outline of the General Relativity Theory, Cambridge University Press.
French, R., 1987. The geometry of visual space. Noûs 21, 115–133.
Gregory, R.L., 1981. Mind in Science. Weidenfeld & Nicholson, London.
Hawking, S., 2001. The Universe in a Nutshell. Bantam Press, London.
Heller, M., 1984. Temporal parts of four dimensional objects. Philos. Stud. 46, 323–334.
Kleiser, R., Seitz, R.J., Kiehelberg, B., 2004. Neural correlates of saccadic suppression in humans. Curr. Biol. 14, 195–197. http://dx.doi.org/10.1016/j.cub.2004.02.036.
Köhler, W., 1947. Gestalt Psychology. Liveright, New York.
Kovács, L., Papathomas, T.V., Yang, M., Fehér, A., 1996. When the brain changes its mind; interocular grouping during binocular rivalry. Proc. Nat. Acad. Sci. U.S.A. 93, 508–511.
Kuhlenbeck, H., 1958. The meaning of "postulational psycho-physical parallelism". Brain 81, 588–603.
Linde, A., 1990. Particle Physics and Inflationary Cosmology. Harwood Academic Publishers, Chur, Switzerland.
Lloyd, G., 1978. Time and existence. Philosophy 53, 215–228.
Penrose, R., 1994. Shadows of the Mind: A Search for the Missing Science of Consciousness. Oxford University Press, Oxford.
Price, H.H., 1953. Survival and the idea of another world. Proc. Soc. Psych. Res. 50, 1–25.
Quine, W.V., 1982. Methods of Logic, fourth ed. Harvard University Press, Cambridge, MA.

Quinton, A.M., 1962. Spaces and times. Philosophy 37, 130–147.

Ramachandran, V.S., Blakeslee, S., 1998. Phantoms in the Brain. Morrow, New York.

Russell, B., 1948. Human Knowledge its Scope and Limits. Allen & Unwin, London.

Schilder, P., 1950. The Image and Appearance of the Human Body. International Universities Press, New York.

Searle, J.R., 1992. The Rediscovery of the Mind. MIT Press, Cambridge, MA.

Smythies, J.R., 1953. The experience and description of the human body. Brain 76, 132–145.

Smythies, J.R., 1959a. The stroboscopic patterns. Part I. The dark phase. Br. J. Psychol. 50, 106–116. http://dx.doi.org/10.1111/j.2044-8295.1959.tb00688.x. Article first published online: April 13, 2011.

Smythies, J.R., 1959b. The stroboscopic patterns. Part II. The phenomenology of the bright phase and after-images. Br. J. Psychol. 50, 305–318.

Smythies, J.R., 1960. The stroboscopic patterns. Part III. Further experiments and discussion. Br. J. Psychol. 51, 247–255. http://dx.doi.org/10.1111/j.2044-8295.1960.tb00747.x. Article first published online: April 13, 2011.

Smythies, J., 1994a. The Walls of Plato's Cave. Avebury, Aldershot.

Smythies, J., 1994b. Requiem for the identity theory. Inquiry 37, 311–329.

Smythies, J., 2009. 'Reality' and 'Virtual Reality' mechanisms in the brain and their significance. J. Conscious. Stud. 16, 69–80.

Smythies, J., 2013. What neuronal activity constitutes the NCCs? J. Conscious. Stud. 20, 196–202.

Smythies, J., 2014. The nature of consciousness and its relation to the brain: the pith of a formidable problem and its possible solution. J. Conscious. Stud. 21, 183–202.

Smythies, J., Doreye, M., 2016. The Brain as a Massively Asynchronous Organ: A New Paradigm in Neuroscience. Submitted.

Smythies, J., Ramachandran, V.S., 1998. An empirical refutation of the direct realist theory of perception. Inquiry 40, 437–438.

Stannard, R., 1987. Making Sense of God's Time. The Times. August 22nd.

Vernon, M.D., 1962. A Further Study of Visual Perception. Cambridge University Press, Cambridge.

Werth, L.F., 1978. Normalizing the paranormal. Am. Philos. Q. 15, 47–56.

Weyl, H., 1949. Philosophy of Mathematics and Natural Science. Princeton Univ. Press.

Yarrow, K., Haggard, P., Heal, R., Brown, P., Rothwell, J.C., 2001. Illusory perceptions of space and time preserve cross-saccadic perceptual continuity. Nature 414, 302–305. http://dx.doi.org/10.1038/35104551.

Zeki, S., May 19, 2015. A massively asynchronous, parallel brain. Philos. Trans. R. Soc. Lond. B Biol. Sci. 370 (1668). http://dx.doi.org/10.1098/rstb.2014.0174. pii: 20140174.

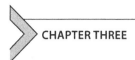

CHAPTER THREE

A Defense of Representational Realism

Robert French

Adjunct Instructor, Philosophy, Oakland Community College, Waterford Township, MI, United States

How is it that when we open our eyes that we are aware of at least what we take to be the front surface of distal physical objects. An obvious issue for the literal defence of this claim is that what links us (light) with these distal objects travels from the distal objects to the eye and not vice versa. How, then, are we supposed to "reach out" to these distal objects so as to directly perceive them?

Various schemes have been invoked by so-called "direct realists" for the creation of these linkages. These purported linkages include, but are not limited to, F. Brentano's (1874/2015, p. 92) sense of intentionality (Smith, 2002), demonstrative reference (Campbell, 2002), rigid designators in possible worlds (Tye, 1995, p. 184), and physical representational states providing information about distal objects of perception (Dretske, 1995, p. 2). However, unlike the case with indirect realism where there is readily available physical explanation for these linkages (the passage of light rays between the distal objects and our eyes), it is incredibly unclear to me as to how any of these proposed mechanisms is to be instantiated.

In any event my answer to the foregoing conundrum is to deny the presupposition that we are immediately aware of even the front surfaces of distal physical objects when, under the attitude of common sense, we claim to see them. Instead I hold that this presupposition is false and that what we take (or better mistake) for the distal front surfaces are in fact phenomenal events in a private phenomenal mental space.

What I hold is responsible for the alleged directedness to the distal object under this account is just the mistaken assumption that this object is, in fact, immediately presented. That this is not what is actually going on I hold should be obvious from such cases of illusions as the Ames rooms and counterrotating trapezoidal window, or viewing so-called 3D movies (where there are phenomenal depth effects in spite of the fact that the

Direct versus Indirect Realism
ISBN 978-0-12-812141-2
https://doi.org/10.1016/B978-0-12-812141-2.00003-9

movie screen is flat) where the physical world appears contrarily different from the way it is. Even for cases not ordinarily classified as illusions, such as viewing the night sky or the daytime blue sky, the nature of the distal object is incredibly different from what is immediately presented visually. In the case of the night sky distal objects exist at very different times and in the case of the blue sky there is not even a fixed distal object. Still for most purposes of ordinary life we get away with mistaking distal objects for the corresponding phenomenal experiences, which is why the attitude of naïve realism works as well as it does. Also, as far as I can see, contra Smith (2002, p. 16), this mistaken identity is sufficient to account for public discourse concerning the distal objects, which are only indirectly perceived.

In this paper I term the foregoing position as "representational realism," which is a traditional term for the theory of perception holding that the perception of distal physical objects is mediated by both the existence and the "apprehension" of an internal state of affairs—a representation of the objects. Note that this is different from the position, which Tye (2000, Ch. 3) calls "representationalism" (whereby it is held that representational states, due to their intentionality, transparently provide direct access to distal physical properties) but my usage predates this. I will confine my remarks to defending representational realism against a series of alleged inconsistencies, which have at least historically been thought by many to be decisive. I am aware that there is a continuing literature on this topic, but these alleged inconsistencies still are often maintained to have some force.

The alleged incoherencies in representational realist positions, which I will be investigating, are the following:

1. Such a theory would result in an infinite perceptual regress either of physical sense system, such as eyes, whereby another perceptual system would be required to sense whatever a first system senses and so on, or of experiences, whereby a second experience would be required to be aware of a first experience and so on;

2. that it holds that perception is "indirect," whereas it is manifestly "direct" in that we "immediately" perceive distal physical objects without the perception being "mediated" by something else;

3. that it will result in the postulation that we are just aware of "pictures" of objects rather than the objects themselves, whereas this is manifestly not the case as is borne out by ordinary perceptual language; and

4. that just to state such a theory of perception, violence must be done to ordinary language inasmuch as ordinary perceptual language does not allow a distinction, which is fundamental to the theory of representational realism, between "perception of objects" and the "objects of perception," to get off the ground.

I will not present any positive arguments for the truth of representational realism, although I have done so elsewhere (French, 1987a,b, 2016), but will instead just try to show why I believe that each of the foregoing alleged incoherencies in the position do not apply if the position is properly understood. While obviously there are many interconnections among these issues, I will still attempt to examine each of them separately, although pointing out at the same time ways in which they each gain at least some of their initial degree of plausibility from the other claims.

1. PERCEPTUAL REGRESS ARGUMENTS

I begin my discussion of perceptual regress arguments by distinguishing among three classes of arguments. Arguments from the first class have been put forward by D. M. Armstrong (1960, p. 9) and J. J. Gibson (1950, p. 54, 1967, p. 226, 1979, p. 60) among others. These arguments claim that if representational realism was to be correct, this, in the case of visual perception, would result in a regress of "eyes" as perceptual systems in that a second eye would be required to "see" what a first eye sees, and that a third eye would be required to "see" what that eye sees and so on indefinitely. Arguments for regresses along similar lines are sometimes given for other senses as well, such as with the claim, with respect to the sense of touch, of the need to posit "homunculi" or "body images" feeling pains in various parts of their "bodies" to explain our perceptions of pains in our own body. Arguments from the second class involve the claim that the cognitive processing, which occurs in perception must invoke a "little man" to interpret the results of the processing, in which case, no genuine progress has been made toward a reduction to nonintentional explanations. An early version of this type of argument was discussed by R. Descartes (1637/1965, p. 101), and more recently D. Dennett (1978) has disputed their validity. The third class of arguments, a notable instance of which was advanced by G. Ryle (1949), involves the claim that if perception involves sensing a "sensum," as representational realism maintains, then this will result in a "phenomenal regress," in that a second sensum will be required to sense the first sensum and that a third sensum will be required in turn to sense it and so on. It may be noted that the logical structure of all three classes of arguments is essentially the same since they all hinge on maintaining that if a perceptual operation be invoked in performing some function in the perceptual process, it will need to be invoked at further stages as well. My attack on the arguments will involve attacking this principle since I hold that once a phase of the perception process has been performed, it will have served its purpose, and hence at least typically there will be no need to repeat it.

Consider first the eye regress argument in the literal sense of "eyes" as being optical systems. Gibson has presented numerous times, as in the following two passages:

> If the retinal image were really a picture there would have to be another eye behind the eye with which to see it. The notion that we see our retinal image is based on some such idea as a little seer sitting in the brain and looking at them. The question that arises is how can he see?
>
> **Gibson (1950, p. 54)**

> But the eye is not a camera in the sense of a device producing a visible image. If it were such a device there would have to be a man to look at the retinal image or a little man in the brain to look at the image 'projected' on the brain. The man would have to have an eye to see the image with, so we are back where we started. Worse off, in fact, for we are faced with the insoluble paradox of an infinite series of nested individuals, each little man looking at the brain of the next bigger man.
>
> **Gibson (1967, p. 228)**

In spite of superficial resemblances, Gibson's points in the two passages are rather different. In the first argument he is arguing against the claim that we see our retinal images, as opposed to distal physical objects, by claiming that this would be analogous to seeing a picture (with the retinal image being the analogue of the picture), whereby something else would be required to see the picture; i.e., a picture of the picture. In Gibson's second argument he tries to show how it is misleading to compare the eye to a camera since there the function is to produce a static image on the film in the back, and if human vision worked like that the question would arise as to how this image itself would be perceived. I will be dealing with the issue as to whether representational realism need be committed to the position that we just immediately perceive "pictures" of distal objects, as opposed to the distal objects themselves, shortly, so for now I will confine my remarks to the issue as to whether our retinal image need require further eyes.

The following critique of Gibson's eye regress arguments bears a fair amount in common with a critique of a similar argument made by Armstrong, which G. Thrane (1977) has presented. To begin my critique, I find it to be useful to consider the issue as to what the function of the eye is. I do not wish to become bogged down here in the dispute between Gibson and various earlier theorists over the purposes and overall functions of visual perception, such as the relative importance of the retinal image actually being an image or whether, as Gibson maintained, the function of the retina instead basically just involves the fovea "picking up," by means of eye movements, information in an array of ambient (reflected) light. I wish to point out though that at least one function of the eye is neutral with respect to such disputes, that being the role of the lens and cornea of the eye in focusing light (changing diverging light cones into converging cones so as to come to points on a surface, in this case, the retina). Now, it can be pointed out that once this focusing operation has been performed, light rays impinging on distinct retinal points will originate from different directions. It can also be seen that this operation is a prerequisite for either the forma- tion of a retinal image or Gibson's notion of information pick-up since both of these require that there be a one-to-one correspondence between the light rays impinging at any given moment at distinct retinal points and the distal origination points (typically points of reflection) of those rays. The issue can be raised then as to why, once such a focusing operation has been performed in the visual perception process, there should be any need to have it be repeated at a later stage, as was implied by the claim that further eyes, as optical systems, would be required there.

This is where the second version of the regress argument starts to possess a certain force since even if it is possible to transfer an image among various projection centers of the brain without refocusing light rays (since no lens need be required in the transferring process), this in no way explains how either visual percepts are generated or how information is processed so that objects can be identified. It should be emphasized that these are distinct problems, although it is still possible that their solutions may bear at least certain features in common. For example, in the case of visual perception operations akin to D. Marr's (1982) 2 1/2 D sketch (a two-dimensional rep- resentation of the visual field where depth information, the "1/2 D," is also included at each point) may both be necessary to account for phenomenal perceptions of visual depth, and also as a crucial step in the determination of objects' three-dimensional shapes from the two-dimensional images; which in turn may be a prerequisite for their linguistic identification. I will now present a few suggestions concerning how regresses can be avoided with respect to both problems, beginning with the identification problem.

To begin my discussion of the identification problem, note that a large amount of evidence has been uncovered showing that the further along the visual perceptual processing chain that signals from the retina progress (i.e., from area 17 to areas 18 and 19 of the visual cortex and subsequently to polysensual "association cortices") it is both the case that neurons only fire for increasingly specific stimuli ranging from edges oriented at specific angles or moving in specific directions in area 17, to edges of specific lengths or "corners" in areas 18 and 19 (Hubel and Wiesel, 2005) to reportedly only faces and hands for certain neurons in the superior temporal sulcus (Bruce et al., 1981), and also that retinal regions, which the neurons are responsible to become increasingly large—ranging from just a few minutes of arc from some of the "simple cells" in area 17 to whole quadrants of the visual field for some neurons in the superior temporal sulcus.

Networks of neurons can in turn be characterized as performing relatively complex functional tasks, such as reconstructing visual depth information from the binocular depth cue of retinal disparity or determining the three-dimensional motion of objects from two-dimensional patterns (see Ullman, 1979). Even here though, individual neurons will still be performing individual tasks (comparable to the relatively simple tasks performed by individual lines of a computer program as compared to the relatively complex task of the whole program), and as Dennett (1978) points out, the smaller the network, the tasks being performed will be progressively "stupider." As Dennett (1987) has also pointed out, the activities of the individual neurons can be described either functionally (as edge detectors for neurons in area 17, or as hand or face identifiers for neurons in the superior temporal sulcus) or mechanistically in terms of the physical properties of the neural circuits. He takes the "intentional stance" involved with the functional explanation just to involve a useful shortcut for predicting behavior and to be completely compatible with a mechanistic description. Since there is no need to posit further mechanistic systems to explain the activities of the neural circuits from a mechanistic perspective, in view of the just-mentioned compatibility of this perspective with a functional one, there would seem to be no need to posit further "homunculi" either to understand the tasks being performed.

I now turn to the problem of the actual generation of visual percepts from neural activity in various projection centers of the brain. As Descartes (1637/1965, p. 101) argues in the following passage from his *Dioptics*, there is no reason for thinking that this occurs by other eyes viewing activity in these centers:

> *Now while this picture (the retinal image), in thus passing into our head, always retains some degree of resemblance to the objects from which it proceeds, we yet need not hold, as I have already sufficiently shown that it is by means of this resemblance that it enables us to perceive them, as if there were again in our brain yet other eyes with which we are able to apprehend it.*

I will not even attempt to provide a positive solution to the mind (in the conscious sense) body problem raised by Descartes, and thus I confine my remarks to making two points. First, it can be remarked that any features discriminated in our phenomenal perceptual fields, such as visual depth, must possess neural counterparts in which the corresponding information is encoded; e.g., a neural correlate for phenomenal visual depth would have to involve a coding of something comparable to Marr's 2 1/2 D sketch. Secondly, I wish to emphasize, in agreement with Descartes, that there is no reason to think that another set of sensory organs (e.g., eyes, in the case of vision) is involved with the causal determination of percepts since that would only lead to a regress.

I now turn to my discussion of the third type of regress argument, the "phenomenal" regress argument. Ryle (1949, p. 213) presents a version of such an argument, in the context of criticizing sense-data theories of perception as follows:

> *The theory says that when a person has a visual sensation, on the occasion, for example, of getting a glimpse of a horse race, his having this sensation consists of his finding or intuiting a sensum, namely a patchwork of colors. But if having a glimpse of a horse-race entails having at least one sensation, then having a glimpse of color patches must again involve having at least one appropriate sensation, which in turn must be analyzed into the sensing of yet an earlier sensum, and so on forever.*

Thus, Ryle argues that representational realism is incoherent since in making the claim that we are never immediately aware of distal physical objects, but instead merely immediately sense something else, sometimes referred to as "sense data," or any of the various synonyms for them (e.g., "qualia," "percepts," "sensations," "sense experiences," etc.), it involves itself in an infinite regress. A regress must occur, he holds, since, just following the logic of the sense-data theory, something else besides an original set of sense data will be required to sense those sense data. I wish to question though why this last step follows, and thus why a regress need develop on this point.

It is important not to be misled by the grammar of our ordinary perceptual vocabulary here. For example, such perception verbs as "see," "perceive,"
and even "sense," are all transitive verbs, and hence their usage would seem,
prima facie, to entail making distinctions between, respectively, the "seer"
and the "seen," the "perceiver" and the "perceived," and the "senser" and
the "sensed." If these distinctions are allowed to be legitimate, then Ryle's
phenomenal regress would follow. In the last portion of my paper though I
will argue that what is really going on here is that the ordinary language of
perception is theory-laden, implicitly assuming the truth of naïve realism,
since under that doctrine what we immediately "see," "perceive," and even
"sense" is physical, and thus the foregoing distinctions make sense. However,
this is not the case if representational realism is correct since under that
doctrine it is claimed that what we are immediately aware of in perception
is phenomenal in character. Thus, representational realism holds that there
is a fundamental difference between requiring sense data for the perception
of a distal stimulus and requiring further sense data to sense "sense data" per
se. This is because it holds that the very existence of sense data, inasmuch
as it is a phenomenal existence, constitutes their being sensed. Thus, it is
also held that the distinction between the "senser" and the "sensed" breaks
down here; i.e., what is "sensed" is held to just be a part of the conscious
mind of the "senser." If this cannot be stated using the ordinary language
of perception, so much the worse for that language; i.e., this just shows its
theory-ladenness.

It can be noted now that a parallel can be drawn between the solution
that I just sketched for the phenomenal regress argument and the solutions that I gave to the literal eye regress arguments. In both cases I have
argued that once a perceptual operation has been performed, its function
has thereby been accomplished, and hence there is no need to repeat it at a
later stage of the perceptual process. Even though the focusing of light by
the eye, the "processing" of information from the retinal images prior to the
creation of visual sensations, and the very existence of these sensations in
the conscious mind, each represents quite distinct stages in the visual perception process, none of them need be repeated in the process, and thus any
purported regresses here can be avoided. This concludes my discussion of
perceptual regress arguments, and thus I will now turn to a discussion of the
next alleged incoherency for the theory of representational realism—the
claim that it makes the perception of distal physical objects be "indirect"
rather than "direct."

2. IS PERCEPTION DIRECT OR INDIRECT?

The subject matter of whether perception is "direct" or "indirect" is a tricky one to resolve since in the literature the words are used in different ways. In particular, it is important to clearly distinguish between an epistemic use of the words, whereby it may be claimed that perception is, respectively, "direct" or "indirect" depending on whether or not it is thought that an inference or a conjecture is involved in the perception process, and a nonepistemic or "ontological" sense, whereby it is claimed that perception is, respectively, "direct" or "indirect" depending on the existence or nonexistence of causal intermediaries (see Cornman, 1972). Holding that perception is "direct" in the epistemic sense can be likened to holding a qualitative identity (in at least some respects) between "representations," "fields of percepts," or any analogues of these and distal physical objects of perception; while holding that perception is "direct" in the ontological sense can be likened to holding a numerical identity here. Disputes over whether perception is "direct" or "indirect" are exacerbated by not clearly distinguishing between these different senses, and this often results in arguments at cross purposes to each other. To make this point using the analogy just given with qualitative and numerical identity, it can be seen that showing that two objects are qualitatively identical in no way also shows that they are numerically identical, and obviously this point can be lost if the distinction is overlooked because we use the same word "identical" to refer to both of these senses. I wish to argue now that an analogous confusion has occurred in the literature in the philosophy of perception by not clearly distinguishing between the analogous two senses of "directly perceive."

Consider the case of Gibson. He has argued that perception is "direct" due to the existence of invariants in the optical arrays impinging on the eyes and the way these invariants are preserved in the subsequent passage of electrical impulses along neural pathways into the central nervous system (Gibson, 1979, Ch. 14). By thus pointing to the presence of causal processes linking distal physical objects being perceived with our central nervous system, it is clear that Gibson held a version of the causal theory of perception. Thus, while his position may be compatible with the claim that perception is "direct" in the epistemic sense, it is clearly not also compatible with its being "direct" in the ontological sense due to the presence of these intervening causal processes in between the distal physical objects being perceived and the perceiver. This raises an issue though concerning the ontological status of the "representations," or their analogues, of the physical objects being perceived, and as far as I can see Gibson has nothing positive to say on this issue, perhaps because he does not distinguish between the two senses of "directly perceive," and thus glosses over the numerical distinction just pointed out. As far as I can see analogous points can also be made concerning Dretske's (1995) account.

It would seem then that a representational realist may or not also be a "direct realist" in the epistemic sense of holding that our knowledge of physical objects is "immediate" in the sense of not being "mediated" by any such fallible intermediaries as conjectures or inferences, and in fact much work has been done in developing "reliability" theories of knowledge in this regard (see Dretske, 1981). There is also considerable evidence though that at least in the case of visual perception the system often makes assumptions such as in the cases of misleading stereopsis as with 3D movies, the phi phenomenon inducing perceived motion, and Ullman's (1979, 1980) example of how assumptions of rigidity are involved with the underdetermination of visual motion from retinal images. In any event, a representational realist cannot also be a "direct realist" in the ontological sense of numerically identifying a distal stimulus with our perception of it since to do so would be to deny that there is anything "representational" about the perception process; i.e., it would collapse the distinction between the "representation" and the "object represented." Thus, representational realism cannot hold that perceptions of distal physical objects are "immediate" in the sense of not being causally mediated by any intervening physical processes; i.e., the passage of light rays and various neural transmissions for the case of visual perception. A representational realist must therefore be prepared to give an account of the ontological status of the "representation" side of the perceptual causal chain since they hold that this is at least numerically distinct from the distal physical objects being "represented," and this is what I see most modern self-styled "direct realists" as having failed to do. In any event, I would like to go on now to make use of some of the preceding points in critically examining the claim that representational realism will require that "pictures" of objects rather than the objects themselves be the "immediate" objects of perception.

3. DO WE SEE "PICTURES" OF OBJECTS OR THE OBJECTS THEMSELVES?

The following points concerning the issue as to whether in any important sense we "see" pictures of distal physical objects rather than the objects themselves if representational realism is correct are closely tied in with both my discussion of the eye regress argument (with respect to the claim that we "see" our retinal images instead of their objects) and also the preceding discussion concerning whether perception is "direct" or "indirect." For example, with respect to this latter issue, it might seem that maintaining that perception is "indirect," in the ontological sense, would entail the position that we do not see physical objects due to their only being "indirectly perceived." It might also seem to follow then that the "direct" or "immediate" object of perception would have to be something else, which would be analogous to a "picture" of the distal objects being "indirectly perceived," in at least the sense of its bearing a "representing" relationship to these objects while being numerically distinct from them. Candidates for what is immediately perceived, and which are thus being likened to "pictures" of the distal objects being "indirectly perceived," would include light reflected from the objects and entering our eyes, our retinal images of the distal objects, even electrical patterns in our visual cortices, and, finally visual percepts themselves. Consider now the following passage where Gibson (1979, p. 147) contrasts his own position of "direct perception" with the just given one of perception being mediated by "pictures" in various senses.

> Direct perception is what one gets from seeing Niagara Falls, say, as distinguished from seeing a picture of it. The latter kind of perception is mediated. So when I assert that perception of the environment is direct, I mean that it is not mediated by retinal pictures, neural pictures, or mental pictures.

I make two distinct points in reply to Gibson—the first is that each of the foregoing candidates for being objects of "immediate perception" are relevantly unlike "pictures" in any literal sense of the word; and the second is that there is something very misleading in our ordinary language talk about "objects of perception," namely that it assumes the truth of naïve realism. To begin my discussion of the first point, it can be pointed out that seeing "pictures," in the literal sense, involves light being reflected from the picture and subsequently entering the eyes. If visual perception worked in this manner it would obviously result in the "eye regress" previously discussed, inasmuch as the perception of a picture, in the literal sense, requires eyes to see it. Thus, the point about just "directly seeing" pictures here must be at least a bit more metaphorical, such as in my previously mentioned claim that representational realism, in making a numerical distinction between perceptions and their objects, is at least implicitly making the claim that perceptions are like pictures in the sense of "representing" their objects while being numerically distinct from them.

The concept of "representation" just alluded to deserves elaboration, at least so as to avoid conflating it with other notions that are sometimes brought in here, notably "resemblance." As N. Goodman (1976, Ch. 1) has rightly emphasized, the "representation" relation between pictures and the physical objects being depicted need not be one of resemblance both because in the case of "abstract" pictures one may be hard pressed to find any properties in common between the two, and since the overriding criteria used in disputes over what objects are being depicted by pictures are typically not ones concerning resemblance but instead causal and intentional facts. For example, pointing out that a portrait is a terrible likeness of a particular person does not establish that a different person was being depicted while showing that the artist was in fact trying to depict someone else would constitute such evidence, and similar points can be made concerning photography and causal connections by means of light rays.

In spite of the foregoing facts, it would seem that at least in the case of "realistic" pictures, the representation relation will at least involve resemblances. In particular, a metric invariant of perspective is the cross-ratio, which for four collinear points $X_1 - X_4$ is $\dfrac{(X_1 - X_2) \times (X_2 - X_3)}{(X_1 - X_4) \times (X_2 - X_4)}$. There are also various topological invariants, ignoring complications when occlusions occur, as whether a figure is open or closed and the number of sides enclosing them. In fact, I do not find Goodman to be sufficiently cognizant of the versatility of some of these invariants; for example, the value of the cross-ratio is independent of both the angle of view and the viewing distance. It would seem then that, if my foregoing analysis of the sense in which Gibson was a "direct realist" is correct, then there need be no conflict between his position and the claim that perception involves apprehending "pictures" in the "metaphorical" sense just elucidated. Gibson has really only argued for a qualitative identify, in certain respects, between perceptions and their distal objects, and this is compatible with perception being ontologically mediated by 'pictures' in the foregoing "metaphorical" sense.

This completes my discussion of the first point—whether or not perception is mediated by "pictures"—which I wished to make. Inasmuch as my second point concerns the theory-ladenness of ordinary perceptual language—in this case concerning what the proper object of perception is—I will make it within the context of my overall discussion of that topic. Thus, I now turn to my argument that representational realism cannot be adequately characterized using the ordinary language of perception due to certain assumptions about the nature of perception made by language per se.

4. THE THEORY-LADENNESS OF ORDINARY PERCEPTUAL LANGUAGE

To begin my discussion of the theory-ladenness of ordinary perceptual language, I wish to point out that it does not allow a distinction, which is crucial to representational realism, between percepts per se and their distal physical objects, to even get off the ground. It is often claimed in this regard (see Ayer, 1940, pp. 19–28 for a phenomenalist version of the position and C. D. Broad (1959, p. 248) for a representational realist version) that ordinary perceptual language is ambiguous concerning what it takes to be the proper object of perception, possessing both a "physical" sense and a "phenomenal" sense, depending on the issue at hand. J. Locke (1690/1959, Bk. 4, Ch. 8, par. 14), for example, speaks of the perception of ideas. Also, Broad (1959, p. 248), argues for the position as follows:

> A result of this is that all words such as 'seeing,' 'hearing,' etc. are ambiguous. They stand sometimes for acts of sensing, whose objects are of course sensa, and sometimes for acts of perceiving, whose objects are supposed to be bits of matter and their sensible qualities. This is especially clear about hearing. We talk of 'hearing a noise' and 'hearing a bell.' In the first case we mean that we are sensing an auditory sensum, with certain attributes of pitch, loudness, quality, etc. In the second case we mean that, in consequence of sensing such a sensum, we judge that a certain physical object exists and is present to our senses. Here the word 'hearing' stands for an act of perceiving. Exactly the same remarks apply to sight. In one sense we see a penny; in another sense we see only a brown sensum.

However, J. L. Austin (1962, p. 99), in criticism of Ayer's version of the foregoing theory, has persuasively argued that in fact there is only one sense of "see" and other perception verbs being used here, and that when we disagree about what is being seen, we are actually disagreeing about what description pertains to the same object. For example, in the context of a disagreement about whether a bright speck seen in a telescope is a star, Austin claims that the image in the 14th mirror of the telescope is a bright speck, that the bright speck is a star and that the star is Sirius, and that thus just one sense of "see" is being used throughout. It might be noted that an equivocation is made on "speck" here though since the "speck" that is the image in the 14th mirror of the telescope is not the same "speck" that is the star. Still, I think that Austin is making a legitimate point in that, in at least typical cases over disputes concerning what is being perceived, the dispute is over the identification of the object of perception and not over, which numerically distinct object it is that is being perceived. Also, the objects of perception ("objects" are sometimes misleading, as in the case of perceiving shadows) here are always taken to be physical, and thus there is something misleading about Broad talking about seeing "sense data."

In spite of agreeing with Austin on the foregoing points concerning ordinary perceptual language being univocal, I do not think that this shows that representational realism is false. Instead, I believe that it just shows that ordinary perceptual language, in its very grammar, is theory-laden, assuming the truth of naïve realism. Consider the grammar of "see" (similar remarks could be made for other perceptual verbs, such as "sense" and "perceive"). First, it can be pointed out that when we claim to see an object, we claim to be immediately (in the ontological sense previously defined) aware of at least a portion of the object, although we do not have to be aware of each part of the complete object—e.g., I can see a book without seeing each of its pages, or as Descartes (1641/1911) points out in *Meditation II*, see a man by just seeing a portion of his clothing. We also hold that what we see here is physical, and that it continues to exist, in the same format when nobody is looking at it. In fact, it can even be noted that if we should ever gain evidence that any of the foregoing conditions were to be false, such as in the case of a hallucination, we would take back the claim of having seen the object. In other words, "see" is what Ryle (1949, p. 238) has called an "achievement word" in the sense that its correct application presupposes the existence of the object, which it is being claimed is being seen. It can be noted now that the fulfillment of the foregoing conditions constitutes the very definition of naïve realism, and thus the question arises as to how an alternative theory of perception, such as representational realism, can make use of the same vocabulary.

The remedy that I would recommend at this point is to rationally reconstruct the ordinary language of perception in two separate directions. Inasmuch as I have just argued that ordinary perceptual language presupposes the truth of naïve realism, it follows that, just to state an alternative theory, a rational reconstruction of the language is necessary. In the case of representational realism rational reconstructions need to be made in two directions since the theory makes crucial use of a distinction, which cannot even be stated by naïve realism, namely the one between perceptions of objects and the objects of perception themselves. Thus, to adequately state the theory of representational realism reconstructions of two distinct perceptual verbs are needed—one, which I term the "phenomenal" reconstruction, to refer to the apprehension of percepts per se; and also one,

which I term the "physical" reconstruction, to refer to the causally mediated perception of physical objects. I see nothing wrong with allowing such
rational reconstructions into our perceptual language since similar rational
reconstructions have occurred in other fields, notably physics. In the case of
physics, a series of words (including "force," "power," "mass," and "energy")
were taken over from ordinary language and given more precise, and, to
some extent, distorted meanings since ordinary language had not provided
a series of such precise concepts "ready-made." Thus, it can be seen that
when a language does not supply a set of ready-made concepts for a developing field, new ones have to be supplied, either by stipulating meanings
for entirely new words or, in these cases, by rationally reconstructing old
ones.

I now close the paper by illustrating how, by using rationally reconstructed concepts from ordinary perceptual language, representational
realism can handle two problems, which were seen to arise earlier in this
paper; namely, the avoidance of the phenomenal regress argument, and
the issue concerning how to determine the proper object of perception. In the case of the phenomenal regress argument, it can be recalled
that the source of the purported regress was that our ordinary language
perceptual verbs are transitive and thus assume at least a numerical distinction between the "perceiver" and what is "perceived." It follows then
that, if a regress is to be avoided here in the "phenomenal" reconstruction
of ordinary perceptual language, the perceptual verbs cannot be transitive. For example, using the "phenomenal" reconstruction, an active voice
equivalent to the passive voice "redness is sensed (or apprehended) in a
particular location in my phenomenal perceptual field" could be given
here, whereby no distinction would be made between the portion of the
senser's phenomenal field in which at a particular time (using the language
of phenomenology) the object is "constituted," and what is "sensed" or
"apprehended" at that time.

While on the topic of color language I might note that even C. L.
Hardin (1988), who persuasively argues that "color" (as the term is ordinarily used) does not correspond with a fixed property of distal objects,
assumes that it is a univocal concept. This may be true for ordinary usage,
but this is only because it assumes the truth of naïve realism. Under the
attitude of representational realism, there is a clear distinction between
phenomenal color (where red, for example, merges into violet while physically they are opposite ends of the physical light spectrum and a spinning
color wheel is perceived as being white) and a variety of physical senses;

e.g., on such issues as whether objects are colored in the dark, which Locke (1690/1959, Bk. 2, Ch. 8, par. 19) held that they are not, whether they are dispositional or occurrent and whether light is colored. Much is clearly context relative here; e.g., contrast discussions of color in a paint store and in a laser lab.

The second issue that arose earlier concerned a controversy over what constituted the proper object of perception. Different answers can be given depending on which rational reconstruction is being used. In the case of the "phenomenal" reconstruction, the objects will obviously be percepts per se, but the situation is not nearly so clear for the "physical" reconstruction. This is because it is not entirely clear as to where along the physical causal chains leading up to our phenomenal experiences to locate the physical objects of perception. Do we identify them with events in our visual cortices, with our retinal images, with patterns of light impinging on our eyes, with the last objects to reflect that light, or what? While the move of identifying the physical objects of perception with the last objects to reflect the light impinging on the corresponding retinal images may sound promising, as we saw with the case of Austin's analysis, there can be problems even for this solution, in particular with mirror images. The clearest treatment of this topic, which I have seen is that given by Dretske (1981), who provides an analysis in terms of information theory, whereby the object of perception is identified with the object given "primary representation" by a perceiver. I will not attempt to summarize that analysis though, but merely note that pragmatic considerations could certainly be relevant in setting up criteria (e.g., what practical purpose would be accomplished by identifying the physical object of perception with either events in our visual cortices or our retinal images?).

It can be pointed out that the foregoing "physical" reconstruction of perceptual language goes against ordinary usage in that we will not be immediately (in the ontological sense) aware of the objects being "perceived." While this feature will be preserved by the "phenomenal" reconstruction, that reconstruction goes against ordinary usage in that objects of perception are no longer interpreted as being physical objects. Thus, neither reconstruction will preserve all of the connotations of ordinary language perception verbs, but I would say that this just shows that, if representational realism is true, the ordinary language concepts are without application in determining what is actually going on with perception, and hence the need for the rational reconstructions.

REFERENCES

Armstrong, D.M., 1960. Berkeley's Theory of Vision. Melbourne University Press, Melbourne.
Austin, J.L., 1962. Sense and Sensibilia. Oxford University Press, Oxford.
Ayer, A.J., 1940. The Foundations of Empirical Knowledge. Macmillan, New York.
Brentano, F., 1879/2015. Psychology from an Empirical Standpoint. Routledge, New York.
Broad, C.D., 1959. Scientific Thought. Littlefield, Adams @ Co., Patterson.
Bruce, C., Desimone, R., Gross, C., 1981. Visual properties of neurons in a polysensory area in superior temporal sulcus. J. Neurophysiol. 46, 369–384.
Cornman, J., 1972. On direct perception. Rev. Metaphys. 26, 38–56.
Campbell, J., 2002. Reference and Consciousness. Oxford University Press, Oxford.
Descartes, R., 1637/1965. Dioptics. In: Discourse on Method, Optics, Geometry & Meteorology. Translated by Paul Olscamp. Bobbs Merrill, Indianapolis.
Descartes, R., 1641/1911. Meditations. In: Haldane, E., Ross, G. (Eds.), The Philosophical Works of Descartes. Cambridge University Press, Cambridge.
Dennett, D., 1978. Brainstorms: Philosophical Essays on Mind and Psychology. Bradford Books, Cambridge.
Dennett, D., 1987. The Intentional Stance. Bradford Books, Cambridge.
Dretske, F., 1981. Knowledge and the Flow of Information. Bradford Books, Cambridge.
Dretske, F., 1995. Naturalizing the Mind. Bradford Books, Cambridge.
French, R., 1987a. The Geometry of Vision and the Mind Body Problem. Peter Lang, New York.
French, R., 1987b. The geometry of visual space. Nous 21, 115–133.
French, R., 2016. Apparent distortions in photography and the geometry of visual space. Topoi 35, 523–529.
Gibson, J.J., 1950. The Perception of the Visual World. Houghton Miffllin, Boston.
Gibson, J.J., 1967. The Senses Considered as Perceptual Systems. Houghton MIfflin, Boston.
Gibson, J.J., 1979. The Ecological Approach to Visual Perception. Houghton MIfflin, Boston.
Goodman, N., 1976. Languages of Art. Hackett Publishing Co., Indianapolis.
Hardin, C.L., 1988. Color for Philosophers. Hackett Publishing Co., Indianapolis.
Hubel, D., Wiesel, T., 2005. Brain and Perception. Oxford University Press, Oxford.
Locke, J., 1690/1959. An Essay Concerning Human Understanding. Dover, New York.
Marr, D., 1982. Vision. W. H. Freeman, San Francisco.
Ryle, G., 1949. The Concept of Mind. Hutchinson's University Library, London.
Smith, A.D., 2002. The Problem of Perception. Harvard University Press, Cambridge.
Thrane, G., 1977. Berkeley's proper object of vision. J. Hist. Ideas 38, 243–260.
Tye, M., 1995. Ten Problems of Consciousness a Representational Theory. MIT Press, Cambridge.
Tye, M., 2000. Consciousness, Color, and Content. MIT Press, Cambridge.
Ullman, S., 1979. The Interpretation of Visual Motion. MIT Press, Cambridge.
Ullman, S., 1980. Against direct perception. Behav. Brain Sci. 3, 373–415.

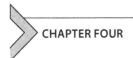

CHAPTER FOUR

Is Direct Realism Falsifiable?

Ernest W. Kent[1,2,3,a]

[1]Formerly: Chief Scientist, Intelligent Systems Division, The National Institute of Standards and Technology, Gaithersburg, MD, United States; [2]Formerly: Director of Research in Information Technology for N. America, Phillips, N.V., Briarcliff Manor, NY, United States; [3]Formerly: Associate Professor of Physiological Psychology and Psychopharmacology, The University of Illinois at Chicago, Chicago, IL, United States

1. INTRODUCTION

Direct Realism is said to entail the "direct" awareness of physical objects without the necessity of any awareness of intervening representations of the objects. I hold that Direct Realism is irrefutable for the reason that to overcome the various objections leveled against it, it has adopted an inherently nonfalsifiable position from which nothing may be deduced over and above what is already contained in the causal chain of intermediate representations of the distal object. In so saying, I refer to modern Direct Realism as distinguished from Naïve Realism (i.e., the position that when we visually view objects we are immediately aware of the front surfaces of the objects being viewed, and these surfaces are both nonmental and continue to exist in the same format when not perceived), which clearly does have falsifiable logical consequences that are not difficult to refute. My belief is that in making concessions to avoid the pitfalls of Naïve Realism, Direct Realism has in the process divested itself of the ability to make any falsifiable statement about perception or to posit a unique falsifiable consequence of the Direct Realist position.

The literature on Direct Realism is large, and there are many variations of the position, some considering one argument, some another, and it is impossible to address them all. Le Morvan (2004) has provided an excellent and lucid summary of the major arguments leveled against Direct Realism, and the logical counterarguments that Direct Realism may make to escape each of them, along with a clear discussion of the distinction between modern Direct Realism and Naïve Realism. I shall therefore take Le Morvan's list of counterarguments as the canonical list of Direct Realist positions for purposes of illustrating the discussion.

My attempt will not be to refute the counterarguments, but to show that in adopting them Direct Realism must in each case give up the ability

[a] Currently Retired

Direct versus Indirect Realism
ISBN 978-0-12-812141-2
https://doi.org/10.1016/B978-0-12-812141-2.00004-0

to provide a logical consequence or falsifiable prediction, and that in sum, they collectively preclude any prediction from Direct Realism as to what will be seen, preclude invalidation of any logical consequence of the Direct Realist position, preclude consideration of any contrary experimental evidence, and hence make Direct Realism nonfalsifiable. I conclude that if all the counterarguments are accepted, Direct Realism has nothing left to say about perception and that it is defined only by the negative assertion that it is "not indirect."

I shall proceed by first proposing *information content* as a unifying way of looking at the distal object and its representations across the physical causal chain, mental states, and conscious awareness. From this perspective I will present a detailed discussion of two of the types of argument Le Morvan addresses (the argument from time delay and the argument from hallucination.) I shall do this by looking at some specific cases and how the Direct Realist position can deal with them, and what the consequences are of doing so. Following this I will review in more general terms the consequences of the entire set of counterarguments.

Information Content—I am referring here to the information inherent in the structure of things, and not, for example, to Shannon's approach, where things are assigned codes based on frequencies of occurrence. This concept of information content will be considered at greater length below.

---

2. PRELIMINARY REMARKS

Much confusion can arise from trying to discuss how mental and physical objects "look" or "appear." These terms are theory-laden, and in many cases can generate confusions as to what is doing the looking, leading to regression arguments. Thinking of sense data that are often assumed to be "pictures in the mind" can lead to differences in understanding what these notions might mean (French, Ch. 3).

It is helpful instead to consider the issue from the perspective of information content because this is something common to both conscious awareness and physical objects and need make no assumptions about what things "look like." By phrasing the issue in terms of the information content of awareness we remain neutral on such issues as whether the object of our awareness is mental or physical. We avoid statements about "seeing things" and similar language that is theory-laden with naïve historical assumptions about how vision works. This also has the advantage of sweeping away confusions such as arise when we speak of "images" in the brain or neural firing patterns not "looking like" the distal objects giving rise to them, as well as various regress arguments. All that is necessary is to explain how it comes to be that there exists some lawful mapping between the information content of my conscious awareness and the information content of the distal object.

This kind of information is inherent in the differential structure of a physical object's properties. It is the kind of information that distinguishes one part of a thing from another and that is embodied in its essence and required for its description, rather than other syntactic usages such as the content of a message or the meaning of a text. This usage is very similar to the concept in Chalmers (1996, Ch. 8). What this means is that things in the physical world have properties that have measures associated with them that have values lying within some range, continuous or discrete, on one or more dimensions. Abstractly they are vector-valued functions on a state space. These values can be represented or "encoded" in the properties of other things through causal interactions with them, and this process may continue through many such stages of representation via causal information flow (cf., e.g., Lizier and Prokopenko, 2010). For example, an object may have the property of differentially reflecting wavelengths of light, and a measure of this property is a value that becomes causally encoded in a change in the mix of wavelengths of light in the wave front reflected from it. This in turn may causally encode the value in differential firing rates of different populations of cones in your retina and so on. Each of these has information content that can be expressed as functions of the property values of their differential structure.

Whether information in this sense supervenes on substance, or vice versa as some have suggested (Wheeler, 1989), it is clear that so far as our conscious experience of things is concerned they are inseparable. Our awareness of things, regardless of what the ontology of our conscious experience may be, unarguably has discriminable parts and hence embodies this sort of information. These differentiated parts have properties that correspond to values that range over multidimensional information spaces. You can, for example, arrange the lightness or darkness of patches in the visual field on a scale of lighter to darker, or place them on the color solid, and then map them into information spaces of properties of the physical object. Our awareness is thus an embodiment of information in the same way as is the physical substance of the distal objects. When we consider the relation between the distal object and awareness in terms of transformations that map this information content from one to the other, we may discuss the lawfulness and veridicality of the mapping without need to discuss ontological differences between "color" as a property of a distal physical object and "color" as a property of a neural firing pattern or "color" as a property of a mental experience. Note that such things as sense data are neither required nor prohibited by this manner of describing the causal chain of intermediate representations. Awareness might supervene directly on neural processes or on intermediate, mind-dependent objects or states.

It is the information content of our awareness that is the important thing presented to our consciousness. There may be some substance or state of being or other thing existing as a ground state of awareness in an undifferentiated field of vision, but it requires to be differentiated to become an awareness of a distal object, and that differentiation is what constitutes instantiation of the information content of the distal object. When we say that our awareness is *of* something we mean that some information from the something has been instantiated in our awareness. "Instantiation" in this case meaning differentially altering the properties of our awareness so as to encode some mapping of transformations between the properties of our awareness and those of the distal object. Thus when we say that our awareness instantiates some information content we are speaking of manipulating awareness itself. In this sense then, the information content of awareness *is* that which is presented to consciousness.

While there are many positions on what constitutes the content of perception, the dispute is over the nature or identity of the stuff that serves as the representation or embodiment of the information presented to awareness, and not the information presented, which simply either does or does not map at least in part through some transformation to the information embodied in the distal object. Indeed, we may have information about the world without awareness, as, for example, in "blindsight," the ability of people who are cortically blind due to lesions in their visual cortex to respond to visual stimuli that they do not consciously see (Weiskrantz, 2007; Sahraiea et. al., 2010), or as in unconscious mental processes. It is difficult, however, even to think of awareness without information, and it may not be a coherent concept. So long as we accept that the information content of our awareness does in fact somehow arise from an external object, the question becomes how and where it is instantiated, and by what means this occurs.

3. DIRECT AND INDIRECT REALISM

I think anyone but a solipsist would agree that there are things that are external to my conscious awareness, and that are not dependent on it, and that information embodied in such things can become part of my conscious awareness. It does not matter for my purpose whether you are pleased to consider the external things to be objects in the sense of Theseus' ship, or arbitrarily circumscribed piles of bosons and leptons; their only necessary feature is that they embody information. Let us call them "objects." "Conscious awareness" is no doubt more contentious, but for my present purposes its only essential property is that it is the embodiment of the information in my consciousness that is influenced by the distal objects. That is, I am not concerned if you care to think of my awareness of the distal object as a mind-dependent thing that is "like" the distal object of my perception by virtue of the information it embodies, or a neural firing pattern that instantiates that information without being "like" it, or the process of becoming aware of it, or the state of being aware of it. All of these, and I believe anything else that anyone might propose to constitute conscious awareness, have in common the property that they embody information determined at least in part by an object external to my consciousness.

In these terms, the difference between Direct and Indirect Realists hinges on the matter of how the instantiation of the information in my conscious awareness is influenced by the information instantiated in the distal object.

It seems to me that the minimal possible meaning of Direct Realism is that

1. by some means information contained in my conscious awareness is determined at least in part by information about the remote object of my perception, and
2. this is accomplished without the cognitive mediation of intervening representations of the information.

I believe the Indirect Realist would accept (1) but deny (2) and wish instead to stipulate:

1a. this is accomplished through transfer of information to my awareness from some intermediate representation of the information, which is the "thing" of which I am cognitively aware.

Then we need to understand what is meant by a "representation." It appears that such things as the image on the retina or neural encodings of that image are commonly meant when reference is made to representations. The essence of representation here is something that instantiates information about the remote object, although perhaps incompletely or in altered form. We can be agnostic on whether the representation is a physical thing or a mental state. Both have information content insofar as they have properties or differential parts.

Direct and Indirect Realists will then differ neither about the fact that information concerning the distal object is somehow embodied in our conscious awareness nor about the fact that our experience entails an awareness of this information but on how that information comes to be embodied in our awareness; that is, whether we are directly or indirectly aware of it.

One additional criterion for our purposes would seem to be that a causal chain exists to account for the transmission of information from the remote object to whatever intermediate representation we are discussing. In the same spirit then, the wave front of light rays passing through any plane en route to the lens of the eye is equally a representation, for it contains all of the information that is contained in the retinal image when those rays have undergone refraction by the lens. This is obvious since we could insert a lens at any point and recover an image of the distal object.

Trivially then, the distal object is not only an embodiment of information but also an exact representation of itself, and its visible surface is a partial representation of itself that participates in the causal chain resulting eventually in the pattern of neural impulses in my brain and so on. Of course the information in that causal chain may undergo transformation or decimation at various points in its career. Modern Direct Realists on the whole seem comfortable with the causal chain, but simply assert that it is *causally* necessary to my perception of the remote object, but not *cognitively* part of that perception (Le Morvan, 2004). It follows from this that they must also be comfortable with the fact that "direct" awareness need not imply *exact* or *complete* awareness since of course the causal chain may involve influences that alter or decimate the information, and generally they seem to accept this as well (Le Morvan, 2004). In particular, differences in our perception in the face of unchanging stimulus conditions, or vice versa, are explained causally, insofar as our understanding of the neurobiology is correct, by differences in neural portions of the causal chains due to influences from learned associations, memory, etc. This is true even in the case of hallucinations as I will discuss below.

Accordingly we suppose that even in these instances the information presented to consciousness is in fact the same or different according to these causal neural factors and that perception even if nonveridical does in fact supervene causally on this information.

The crucial difference then seems to be whether conscious awareness is awareness of the remote object itself or of some one or more of these intermediate causal representations. We may wish to make one minor additional requirement since the object of which the Direct Realist asserts he is directly aware is itself an intermediate representation in the chain causally determining his conscious awareness because the causal chain extends further back to, for example, the light source illuminating it. We should thus probably stipulate that the distal object of direct awareness is understood to be the first link in the causal chain at which information about the distal object enters the chain.

4. THE ARGUMENT FROM TIME DELAY: A THOUGHT EXPERIMENT

We may ask if it is possible to manipulate the information passing along this causal chain in such a way as to distinguish in our awareness between direct awareness of the distal object and awareness of an intermediate representation. Consider the following thought experiment. A clock is placed one light-hour distant from me (it is either a very large clock or I have a telescope, so I can see it). I have an assistant stationed beside the clock, and another stationed 30 light minutes between me and the clock. I am watching the clock as it approaches noon, clock time, at which instant I am still perceiving it to read 11:00 a.m. due to the light-speed limitation on transmission of information. At 12:05, clock time, my first assistant destroys the clock. Later, at 12:30, clock time, my second assistant inserts a red filter in the path of the light rays from the clock to my eye, thereby decimating the information from the clock by removing from it information contained in shorter-wavelength light rays. Thus, at 1:00 p.m., clock time, I see the clock strike noon and appear to turn red, and at 1:05, clock time, it disappears (Illustration 4.1).

What I have now done is to tag a particular subset of intermediate representations of the clock; namely, all the ones subsequent to the placement of the filter. I have tagged them by removing a certain portion of the information about the clock (that contained in the shorter wavelengths) in such a way that they can be distinguished in my conscious awareness, should they enter it. These are simply the original representations of the information from the clock in the causal chain as decimated at an intermediate time to remove

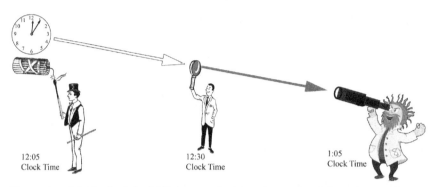

Illustration 4.1 The "red clock" (light gray clock in print versions) thought experiment.

information about its blue–green aspects. These representations physically exist in the wave front of light immediately following the filter, and in all subsequent representations, including my retinal image, the encoding of the image in my neurons, etc. All of these intermediate representations have in common that they did not exist at any time at which the clock existed.

4.1 Arguments From the Experiment

Since with the filter in place I perceive the clock as red, the Indirect Realist can assert that it must be the case that my conscious awareness is of one or more of these tagged representations because at any time either (1) the clock existed, but the causal chain leading to my perception of a red hue did not, or (2) the causal chain of reddened representations existed, but the clock did not. Thus I cannot have conscious awareness of a clock appearing red unless I am having it mediated consciously as well as causally by one of the tagged intermediate representations of the clock. Direct Realists, however, claim that my perception of a clock at a time at which it does not exist is not problematic since Direct Realism does not stipulate that I cannot now be aware directly of something as it was at some time in the past when it did exist (Le Morvan, 2004). Indeed, all of our awareness of things other than possibly our own brain states is an awareness of them as they were at a (possibly very short) past time (Le Morvan, 2004). Although the clock was of course never red and hence not red at that past time, the Direct Realist can further assert that something *appearing* red need not imply that I am aware of a red thing. Thus the Direct Realist may assert that I am aware of a clock in the past appearing red to me (Le Morvan, 2004).

It cannot be argued, however, that my awareness is directly of the clock at a time when it did exist, and in addition a direct awareness of a later event, i.e., the removal of some information about the clock from its intermediate representation, for this destroys the argument that I am causally but not consciously aware of the intermediate representation. Moreover, my conscious awareness must be of the clock appearing red and not an awareness of the clock conflated with direct awareness of an abstract conscious "reddening" event at a later time when the clock did not exist because if the clock is absent there is no such awareness of a "reddening." At the physical level of course there cannot be an "event" consisting of the removal of information that does not exist, and so absent the intermediate representation of the clock there is nothing of which to be aware. This is obvious since no red experience persists when the clock disappears at 1:05 clock time and the filter is still in place.

Alternatively if the filter is placed at 12:40 clock time when the final representation of the clock in the wave front has passed, the clock never appears to turn red but simply persists as it was until it disappears even though the filter is in place.

The Direct Realist then may respond that my awareness is directly of the nonred clock as it was at an earlier time when it existed and that the appearance of redness is the causal but not cognitive result of the causal chain leading from the clock at that time through the filter since Direct Realism does not require that objects appear as they are (Le Morvan, 2004).

Unfortunately what exactly is entailed by "direct awareness of a thing as it was in the past" is not clearly defined, probably has different meanings to different people using the phrase and may be incapable of clear definition until a theory explaining direct awareness is proposed. We might ask if we are to believe that the past things of which we are to be aware still exist in some sense in the past (as in being space-time events in a relativistic block universe) or if we are to understand that they do not still exist in any sense, but we are yet somehow directly aware of their properties as they were when they did exist. If so, in what sense do we understand that those properties or aspects exist?

When does our own awareness of the distal object exist? Does it exist in the past with the object or in the now? The present thought experiment does allow us to argue with respect to this latter question that, in the case that my awareness is direct, we may rule out that my awareness of the clock exists in the past at a time that the clock exists:

1. The clock did not exist at the time of my conscious awareness of a clock appearing red.

2. Therefore if my awareness is of the clock and is not indirect it must either be an awareness of the clock *at* a time in the past or an awareness of the clock *as it was* at a time in the past, but in either case appearing to me nonveridically to be red.

3. By assumption, the causal chain causally determines the content of my conscious awareness including the appearance of redness.

4. At any earlier time at which the clock did exist the red links in the causal chain did not.

5. Therefore if my conscious awareness is *at* an earlier time and directly of the clock appearing red, the causal chain is acting backward in time to make it appear red.

Assuming we reject backward causation we thus conclude that my awareness must be in the now, or at least subsequent to the insertion of the filter (or any other discriminable data decimation event, which may be arbitrarily close to now) while the clock is in the past and never coexists with my awareness. Thus, my awareness in the present must be of the clock *as it was* at a time in the past and not *of* the clock *at* that time in the past. Clearly the same argument applies also to any intermediate representation of the information in the causal chain existing in the past as well as to the clock itself.

What does this imply for the causal chain of representations? Causal links take time to propagate, so if my awareness depends causally on the chain of intermediate representations, then the information content of my awareness in the now must be the end result of this chain and hence my awareness, which instantiates these data, is itself the final link in a causal chain of intermediate representations.

Now if it is asserted that nonetheless the information content of my cognitive awareness is *causally* but not *cognitively* determined by the causal chain of intermediate representations, can the distal object be the direct source of my cognitive awareness?

1. My cognitive awareness of the clock appearing red is in the now.

2. The information content of my awareness in the now is exactly the information about the distal object presented to my consciousness as the perceptible structure of my awareness.

3. None of this information can be numerically identical with any information content of the clock since no aspect of my present awareness in the now, whether information or "something else" can be numerically identical with any part of the clock in the past, so the distinction between them is absolute, and

4. If my awareness and the clock are not at least partially isomorphically colocated, the information in my awareness cannot contain information about the clock contemporaneous with the clock (due to the finite speed of information transmission), and my awareness in the present cannot be colocated with a distal object that does not exist in the present.

5. Therefore the information content of my cognitive awareness cannot be of the clock directly but must be of some later representation.

By this argument we can assert the numerical identity of the information content of my cognitive awareness and the information content of the final link of the causal chain. This reasoning asserts that my awareness is *both* the causal and cognitive result of the causal chain of intermediate representations.

If the information content of my present awareness is thus an awareness of the final representation in the causal chain, is there any sense in which awareness still could be said to be "direct" despite this? One might argue that there is some sense in which "direct" could mean an awareness of the object that was not synonymous with awareness of information about it, but it is not clear that there is any coherent manner in which such a statement could be interpreted.

Irreducibilist Direct Realism, a more interesting possibility from the Direct Realist position, holds that direct awareness is a relation between awareness and the distal object that is not ontologically reducible. Allston (1999) provides an interesting example. To avoid the obvious lack of connection of such a proposal to real events, Allston, like others, admits a *causal* connection between awareness and neural states. To preserve ontological irreducibility he stipulates that the supervenience of awareness on the neurobiology is nomological. This may preserve ontological irreducibility, but it does not protect his position from the argument of the above thought experiment for nomological supervenience is quite good enough to make the argument, and the position advocated here does not depend on the ontological status, provided only that things have parts with discriminable properties. He does not provide much detail on the "relation," but it appears to be essentially the same thing as the mapping discussed above from information content of awareness to information content of the distal object. Thus, aside from the assertion of nomological supervenience, which might some day be vulnerable to disproof, it adds no unique consequences of assuming an ontologically irreducible relation over and above what is explained, within the limits of our understanding of physics and neurobiology, by the causal chain of intermediate representations that it accepts. It thus is nonfalsifiable.

Another avenue open to Direct Realists is to assert that even if in the present experiment awareness is indirect that does not prove that it is in all cases. This is similar to various disjunctivist positions (Byrne and Logue, 2009) and is similarly nonfalsifiable. However, since the present thought experiment is similar in principle to any situation (such as atmospheric absorption) in which a loss of information occurs and is detectable in consciousness, it must be said that such an argument leaves the Direct Realist with very few cases in which to assert that Direct Realism applies.

Any other interpretation of "direct" would seem to require that in some fashion the distinction between my present awareness and the past clock could be collapsed. If this is not some species of crypto-phenomenalism, then there needs be *some* identity, influence, correspondence, or effect other than the causal chain relating my awareness to the distal object to provide substance to the use of "direct." However, any such attempt runs afoul of the fact that there exists no known, nonmystical means for any *direct* influence between the clock in the past and my awareness in the present, which is exactly the reason that Direct Realism accepts the causal chain at the expense of falsifiability.

I can thus think of no falsifiable argument from Direct Realism that can escape the argument from the thought experiment. Suppose, however, that some flaw is found in the reasoning from the thought experiment and that it cannot after all be proven from it that awareness must be the *cognitive* end product of the causal chain of intermediate representations in this case. It still stands that to make it possible that the cognitive awareness is direct in this case, the Direct Realist has had to (1) take refuge in the assertion that the awareness is of the clock as it was at a time in the past, which can only be possible by causal information transmission through the intermediate representations, and (2) agree that the clock can still appear red since Direct Realism need not hold that things appear as they are, while the only available mechanism for this appearance is again the operation of the causal chain of intermediate representations. Thus the asserted "directness" of the awareness is just an assertion, which adds nothing whatsoever over and above what is already given by the intermediate representations and *per se* has no consequences and is thus not falsifiable.

5. HALLUCINATION AND NECESSITY

The argument from hallucination is one of the standard ones leveled at Direct Realism. Obviously we cannot be *directly* aware of objects that do not now and never have existed, as in hallucination, and modern Direct Realists seem to accept this (Le Morvan, 2004). I turn now to the argument from hallucination, and I will do this first by way of considering if Direct Realism is either necessary or sufficient for perception.

If Indirect Realism is correct, then it should be the case that the intermediate representations are both necessary and sufficient for my awareness of a remote object, while direct awareness is neither sufficient nor necessary. The first part is simple; it is generally conceded that the causal chain of intermediate representations is necessary for awareness of distal objects, and any operation that interrupts it results in loss of awareness. Hence direct awareness is not sufficient in the absence of the causal chain of indirect representations.

Can we also show that the intermediate representations are sufficient in the absence of direct awareness, in which case direct awareness is not necessary? This is more difficult but consider the case of hallucinations. Hallucinations do have causal chains and intermediate representations. It is well known that various physical, neurological interventions such as electrical brain stimulation will produce hallucinations ranging from simple sensory experiences to complex perceptions of states of affairs in the external world, depending on the area of the brain targeted. Similarly, a variety of neuropharmacological interventions such as hallucinogenic drugs may be used to alter the neural activity in specific neurochemical pathways resulting in manifest hallucinations of great complexity. In these cases we may say that the causal chain runs from the experimental manipulations through the establishment of particular neural firing patterns in higher levels of the nervous system and into awareness in much the same way as it does when such neural firing patterns are causally produced by ordinary activity in the sensory systems. Again, small, irritative brain lesions in particular areas are found to produce hallucinations, while large lesions of the same areas eliminate such hallucinations (Block, 2012; Collerton, 2014), again suggesting that hallucinations do have neural representations just as ordinary sensory events do. Since there is no external object of which to be directly aware in this case it may be argued that the causal chain is sufficient and that direct awareness is not necessary.

A possible counter to this line of reasoning, however, would be to turn the situation on its head and claim that the neural firing pattern itself was the distal object of which we were directly aware and that the supposed hallucination in the external world was its appearance in conscious awareness and could be so by direct awareness since, "objects need not appear as they really are," (Le Morvan, 2004). This of course is simply to deny that the situation is a hallucination in the first place, so the argument is indeterminate.

We can, however, demonstrate an example of a case that is more difficult to define away in this manner. The nervous system massively decimates the information received from the retina. The information arriving at the retina contains a great deal of redundancy. It is inefficient in terms of biological resources and processing capacity to deal with redundant information. Regions of low variance spatially or temporally are highly redundant since adjacent points can be predicted from boundary regions. Thus the nervous system has evolved mechanisms for discarding information from areas that are spatially or temporally homogeneous and forwarding for subsequent processing only information from spatial or temporal boundaries. This is well known from, for example, work on stabilized images (Pritchard, 1962) and "edge detectors" in the neural visual apparatus (Hubel and Wiesel, 1962; Ewert, 1985; Wilson and Keil, 2001).

The point of interest here is that it can be demonstrated that (1) we are not consciously aware of the *actual* content of spatially or temporally homogeneous image regions, but (2) we do, nonetheless, have conscious awareness of *something* in these areas. An illustrative example is the *Krauskopf effect* (Krauskopof, 1963), in which the subject is presented with a green disk superimposed on a larger, orange disk. Image stabilization techniques are then applied only to the boundary between the orange and green regions. As a result the green disk, which is unchanged on the retina, disappears from our awareness and is replaced in the subject's awareness by a uniform orange region. (It is not necessary to use a stabilized boundary. There are variations of the effect in which the boundary transition is simply made so gradual that the nervous system treats it as a nonboundary region.) This result is interpreted as an example of the nervous system dealing with redundancy through *predictive coding* (Huang and Rao, 2011) in which only spatial or temporal boundaries are processed, and regions between them are inferred from the boundary conditions. These inferences are then an efficient way in which to encode representations of large homogeneous areas in the brain's internal model of the world. It is another example of the general "filling-in" approach in neural representation (Komatsu, 2006; Motoyosh, 1999; Ramachandran and Gregory, 1991). Abnormalities of predictive coding have also been suggested as causes of hallucination in mental disorder (Horga et al., 2014).

In everyday life this works very well most of the time, but the operation of the process can be exposed by unusual circumstances such as the laboratory setup of the Krauskopf effect. Numerous demonstrations of similar phenomena with the same interpretation are available, including higher-level processing such as extrapolation of patterns between stabilized pattern boundaries. In a similar manner, a small object centered in the blind spot disappears, but the area does not appear blank. Rather, it appears as a continuation of whatever surrounds the object in the visual field (Komatsu et al., 2000; Durgin et al., 1995; Spillmanna et al., 2006).

Assuming that our understanding of the neurobiology involved is correct, at least in general outline, it is clear that (1) the nervous system discards the information contained in the causal chain beginning in the green region of the object and ending in its representation in the image on the retina, and (2) it replaces this with a more efficient internal representation of this area of the image based (erroneously in the stabilized case) on information computed and interpolated from other image regions. We have then that, so far as the physical causal chain is involved, the neural representation of the green region of the object is not derived from the green region of the object, but rather is computed from information originating in a different location.

A causal intermediate representation for the region thus exists in the neural apparatus, but it is inherently nonveridical. No orange central region of the distal object exists but one is seen. So far as the causal chain is concerned the intermediate representation is the representation of the central region and not, for example, of something else obscuring it. It is just the way that region is represented and *is* the causal representation of that region appearing in awareness. Moreover the stabilization experiment merely reveals the process; in point of fact it is in operation in the ordinary case when we see the region as green, although not obviously so. Thus we are not seeing something that is obscuring what is really there we are seeing something, which is not there. Since the neural representation is a causally intermediate representation, we cannot say this time that it is the object of which we are directly aware without accepting Indirect Realism. There can be no direct awareness of a nonexistent green central region and we infer that direct awareness is not necessary to conscious awareness.

As a thought experiment, it seems clear that we could even substitute empty space for the central region and stabilize or gradualize the boundary between something and nothing, and we would yet see something. I am not aware of anyone having performed this version of the experiment, but obviously we could and there seems little doubt about the outcome. This would surely qualify as a hallucination for we have conscious awareness of something that is not there yet the intermediate representation is surely a link in the causal representation of that area. In this instance then clearly there could be no direct awareness of the nonexistent central region, and we infer again that direct awareness is not necessary to conscious awareness.

The Direct Realist defense against hallucination, however, is usually some variant of disjunctivism or what amounts to the same thing more elegantly stated, we have, "… no compelling reason to suppose that the objects of awareness in hallucination and in (veridical) perception are ontologically of the same category…," (Le Morvan, 2004). These positions, however, offer no means of predicting (or even of knowing) what experiences of conscious awareness are or are not supposedly "direct," and amount to simply saying, "it's direct unless it's not," a position with no logical consequences, which is seemingly nonfalsifiable. This escapes the issue by asserting that, "…if we suppose for the sake of argument that sense-data (or ideas or the like) are the objects of immediate awareness in cases of hallucination, we need not accept that they are *also* the objects of immediate awareness in (veridical) perception." (Le Morvan, 2004) (I assume that this would also include intermediate neural representations as the objects of immediate experience.) This of course is nonfalsifiable. However, the present example points out that hallucination is a part of our ordinary everyday perceptual experience. The experimental manipulations of the Krauskopf effect only make manifest the fact that interiors of nearly uniform content are constructed in our perception not from their own appearance but from their boundary information. The fact that this works very well in most cases in approximating veridical data does not mean that it is the less hallucination. Thus by appeal to the above defense, the Direct Realist gives up on most of our normal visual interaction with the world.

What is happening causally is just a low-level process thought to be part of a general principle that the nervous system maintains internal models of the world from which it continually generates expectations about the next state of the sensors. Comparison of the expectation with the actual input then permits rejection of noise and updating of the internal model as inputs vary over time. We say that the model is "servoed" to the incoming data. In the case where there is nothing there in the input, the model's best guess is a continuation of the surrounding region and so it uses that to present to other processes (presumably including our awareness) as well as to generate further expectancies until such time as incoming data contradict it. It is of course more complex than this, involving neural versions of Kalman filtering and other refinements, but the idea is that the brain has evolved fundamentally as a control system for the organism, and the control of behavioral output is servoed to the internal model just as the model is servoed to the incoming information. This approach is also used in most modern control systems as well for the same reasons of computational efficiency, missing information, and noise rejection. For an introduction to the ideas involved, see Kent and Albus (1984), and Smythies and d'Oreye de Lantremange (2016). Further perspectives on internal models can be found in Koenderink and van Doorn (1975, 1979), Gordon et al. (2011), Rao (1999), Wolpert et al. (1995), Hohwy (2012), Flach (1990) and Cotterill (1996). Such control-theoretic considerations can be used to explain a great many illusions such as the "Mach Strip" (see Appendix A) perceptual constancies, and in particular the large role that motor functions and feedback from proprioception and kinesthetic sense plays in determining how we perceive the three-dimensional world. It appears in fact that only a small percentage of the information reaching the retina reaches conscious awareness; the majority is provided from the model servoed to that data and comes from stored information or computations similar to those used in information compression techniques for digital television (Smythies and d'Oreye de Lantremange, 2016).

6. DIRECT REALISM HAS NO CLOTHES

Much attention has been directed to considering the epistemological consequences of direct versus indirect awareness, but far less to explaining what "direct" or "immediate" might actually mean. There is not much of a concrete nature concerning what "direct" entails, how it works, what unique consequences or empirical predictions the theory might have, and the like. When we are thus left to a general sense of what "direct" and "immediate" might mean, we arrive at Naïve Realism and a variety of objections that can be based on it. Le Morvan's counterarguments then take the form of stipulating what Direct Realism is *not*.

The Indirect Realist position invokes a causal chain of intermediate representations to account for the appearance of things. This account has developed over time as our understanding of electromagnetic radiation, optics, neurobiology, psychology, control theory, information technology, and other relevant disciplines has deepened. It offers an explanation of many complex aspects of perception, in particular the many ways in which our perceptions differ from our physical models of the external world. The Direct Realist position also relies on this causal chain of intermediate representations to account for all the differences between what we believe to be the true nature of objects and how they appear to us, but in addition asserts that nonetheless our awareness of the objects of perception is in some sense "direct" or "immediate." I believe that when that which Direct Realism is *not* is removed from the possible meanings of "direct," there is nothing remaining over and above the mechanisms of Indirect Realism but a new label.

As a group, Le Morvan's counterarguments are logical and perhaps many if not all are irrefutable. What is striking, however, is that to avoid a potential criticism of Direct Realism each counterargument requires Direct Realism to give up some ability to make a positive assertion about awareness that is falsifiable or that differs in any consequential way from the Indirect Realist position.

Additionally, many of them also require us to adopt beliefs, such as the belief that we can be directly aware of objects that no longer exist, which seem contrary to common sense. Failing to accord with common sense is certainly not fatal, but we would like to have some reason to accept propositions that require it. I believe that on the contrary, Direct Realism *per se* (that is, those aspects of it which differ from Indirect Realism) to avoid the strong criticisms directed against Naïve Realism has had to place itself in the position of making no falsifiable assertions attributable to awareness being "direct." To see this, let us examine the consequences of the counterarguments Le Morvan provides to some of the more important criticisms.

One criticism leveled against Direct Realism is that if our awareness has direct access to a distal object we would expect to be aware of it exactly as it is. Obviously we are not, and to avoid this problem it is asserted as a counterargument that, "Holding that perception of physical objects or events is direct or immediate does not entail that one must also hold that perceived objects or events always appear exactly as they are." This assertion figures prominently in Le Morvan's differentiation of modern Direct Realism from Naïve Realism, which it is asserted holds that objects do so appear, and also figures prominently in several of the later counterarguments. Surely we are then entitled to ask what modern Direct Realism has to say about how objects *are* expected to appear, and why. All that is forthcoming, however, is an appeal to the nature of the causal chain of intermediate representations posited to be the objects of awareness by the Indirect Realists. Nothing to do with "directness" plays any role.

In a similar vein, the criticism is made that awareness cannot be direct because anything that interrupts the causal chain of intermediate representations removes the distal object from our awareness. The counterargument, similar to the one above, is that indeed the intermediate representations are necessary to awareness of the distal object, but only in a causal sense, and that cognitively we are yet directly aware of the object. We would then like to know what should compel us to suppose this, as it seems at first glance to be simply an arbitrary assertion. We would like to ask what logical consequence such a position has or what falsifiable prediction it makes. I cannot think of a way to refute the possibility that there is some sense in which awareness is direct despite its causal dependence on intermediate representations, but only because it is not easy to refute an argument that has no stated consequences. The cognitive directness so salvaged seems devoid of content and generates no falsifiable propositions. This is in contrast to the Indirect Realist position, which would obviously fall if elimination of the intermediate representations failed to alter or eliminate awareness.

A very similar criticism is the "Partial Character of Perception Argument," which asks why, if we are directly aware of an object, we are only directly aware of some parts of it. In the defense against this argument, it is stated that Direct Realism may employ a meaning of "direct" that does not require that all parts of an object be perceived at once. This is certainly true, but we are entitled to ask "what determines which parts we see?" A more complete statement, however, would be that any such meaning of "direct" must be limited to *exactly* those portions of the distal object about which physical information is currently available to the perceiver via intermediate representations. This makes it evident that in fact it is simply a restatement of the restriction of "direct" employed in the defense against the causal argument. It is thus a third instance in which "direct" is simply a label that provides neither explanation nor any further information beyond that also inherent in the indirect position, of which the direct argument now makes use as *causal indirection*. Again the "direct" argument reduces to the simple assertion that the perception is to be called direct, with no suggestion of what that might mean or how it is to be distinguished from indirect perception. Again, it is logically irrefutable for, unlike Naïve Realism, it has no apparent consequences and makes no falsifiable statements.

I have discussed in some detail earlier a particular case of the "Time-Delay Argument," which criticizes Direct Realism on the grounds that because of physical limits on speed of information transmission we do not perceive objects as they are at the time of our awareness, and indeed may perceive objects that no longer exist. Here we may look at the argument in a more general sense, which asks what can "direct" mean if not "as it is now?"

The counterargument begins from the previous position that perception is *causally* indirect, and it is again this that accounts for what we see. It is then maintained that this does not contradict Direct Realism since the concept does not exclude direct perception of objects in the past. (It seems necessary to accept also that this direct perception of past objects is limited to that particular moment in the past corresponding to the moment at which the information currently reaching us left the distal object. If this were not so we might perceive objects before information of them reached us or after it was no longer contemporary with us, which does not occur.) Thus we may ask what additional propositions are made by asserting that we are aware of an object in the past "directly."

The situation is very similar to the previous case. I have a perception of a distal object, which corresponds to the time and nature of information reaching me now, and which is fully explained by this information, including its modifications such as red-shifts and partial losses of information in transit. I am asked to believe, however, that my awareness is a "direct" awareness of an object as it was at some time in the past, modified nonetheless by these causal intermediates *at many different subsequent times*. I am asked to believe this for no other apparent reason than that the statement is not logically self-contradictory. It is clear, however, that the statement is also content-free, for when I am told that my perception is a modified "direct" awareness of an object as it was in the past to escape the argument against Direct Realism that there is no distal object of which to be "directly" aware, I have no more understanding of what "direct" means than before since no meaning other than its use as a label distinguishes it. It has no consequences to distinguish it from the Indirect Realist position, which has some very specific and falsifiable consequences, and in this case as in the preceding arguments reliance must be made on the causal chain of intermediary representations to explain what is in fact seen.

The "Argument from Perceptual Relativity" and the "Argument From Illusion" are closely related. Both entail the criticism that how things appear to us does not necessarily correspond to our beliefs about their actual physical properties (such as shape, for example.). The Direct Realist must explain how this comes about if our awareness is "direct."

The groundwork for the counterargument has already been laid by the assertion that Direct Realism is distinguished from Naïve Realism in that it does not require that objects appear "exactly as they are." There are some very serious problems inherent in understanding what "exactly as they are" might mean, but let us assume for the sake of argument that it is coherent and examine how this position is used. The argument is that it is not necessary to assume that, "if something *appears* F to subject S, then S must be immediately aware of something that *is* F." In other words, there is no necessary connection between distal object and perception implied by the assumption of Direct Realism, *per se*. This saves Direct Realism as so-defined from the problem encountered by Naïve Realism but at the expense of yet another consequence of Direct Realism.

Of course it is acknowledged that there are lawful relations between how things are and how they appear (*e.g.*, the example given is a circular coin appearing as an ellipse when viewed obliquely.) This is explained by asserting that *causally* indirect effects result in intermediate representations, which account for the perception differing from the distal object, but that the perception itself may nonetheless be direct. So we have as before that without appeal to the information transferred to awareness as modified and selected in intervening representations, Direct Realism stands mute on what the perception might be. Yet we are to think that there is some meaningful sense in which the perception is "direct." Each of these steps in the transmission and modification of information is an intervening representation, a "tertium quid," yet we are supposed to think that despite their being acknowledged as causally necessary for the perception, there must be some other unspecified something that is essential and which is provided by the fact of the perception being "direct." This cannot be refuted, for it provides nothing to refute.

The "Argument from Hallucination" has also been discussed above with respect to some specific instances. In general terms the argument is that there are cases where one is aware of something that does not exist, so awareness in these cases cannot be directly of what is seen and must be of some other *tertium quid,* and then, if so in these cases, why not in all? The principle counterargument given is that, "…even if we suppose for the sake of argument that sense-data (or ideas or the like) are the objects of immediate awareness in cases of hallucination, we need not accept that they are *also* the objects of immediate awareness in (veridical) perception." In other words, the defense is essentially disjunctivist and tells us that awareness is direct except when it's not. Once again the defense appears to require a retreat into an inherently nonfalsifiable position. As mentioned in an earlier section the current understanding of neurobiological mechanisms of "filling in" seem to indicate that "it's not" most of the time, but no matter how many specific cases we could demonstrate where it's not direct, it is nonfalsifiable that there might remain instances where it is.

There are some additional counterarguments discussed that I will not deal with here inasmuch as they follow essentially the same line, and I do not think the criticisms they are designed to address are particularly strong in any case.

If we examine the net effect of these considerations, it appears that a Direct Realist position not having the weaknesses of Naïve Realism is in fact no position at all. If one takes seriously that all of the concessions made by Le Morvan's counterarguments are necessary to avoid one or another fatal criticisms, then it seems that indeed Direct Realism can no longer postulate *any* discoverable relationship between awareness and an external world other than that already available from physics, neurobiology, and psychology based on intermediate representations tied together by causal chains. As such Direct Realism is not a unique position on the relation of awareness to the external world because it is content-free in that regard.

We have now that Direct Realism *per se* posits an unexplained connection between awareness and objects in a real, external world, which need not entail any similarity between them, need not be consistent over time nor between individuals, is indistinguishable from experiences admitted to have no connection to external reality, need not have any consistent causal relations with them, are or are not dependent on intervening physical variables, and need not be related to anything that exists at the time of the perceptual event. I do not see how this can be summarized other than by saying that there is no fixed or necessary relationship at all between perceptual events and external objects. If this is what is left of Direct Realism after it is modified to avoid the criticisms of Naïve Realism, what exactly is it? If I say to you that there is good empirical evidence for believing awareness to be based on a dynamic model of the environment maintained by the brain including the neurobiology of the "filling in" phenomenon, neural mechanisms of modeling of motion, and neural mechanisms underlying production of dreams, and you respond, "Yes, all true, but the awareness is nonetheless of the world directly," what precisely is entailed by your statement?

7. SUMMARY

I offered the premise that Direct Realism is nonfalsifiable and has no logical consequences if it adopts the positions required to defend itself against the arguments made against Naïve Realism and took Le Morvan's presentation of counterarguments as a canonical list of Direct Realism arguments for purposes of discussion.

I argued for an approach that focuses on the information content inherent in the structure of both physical objects and conscious awareness to avoid difficulties that arise when speaking of how things "look" or "appear" and which avoids some of the ontological issues of attempting to compare such concepts between the distal object and its representations across the physical causal chain, mental states, and conscious awareness.

I considered two of the arguments, the argument from time delay and the argument from hallucination, in some detail, showing how I would attempt to make them and what the Direct Realist counterarguments would entail. The "red clock experiment" tries to show that awareness must be in the now and of the clock as it was, and not of the clock at an earlier time. From this it argues that awareness in the now must then itself be a representation of information in the now about the distal object and that information in the now cannot be directly from the distal object, hence awareness either is itself the final representation in the causal chain or is an awareness of the final representation. I discussed ways Direct Realism might evade this conclusion and argued that they are nonfalsifiable.

I discussed the neurophysiology of hallucination and that hallucinations have brain-state counterparts and that the nonveridical apparent distal objects are perceptions of these intermediate brain states. A Direct Realist response can be made that the brain states are themselves the distal objects and that the apparent external objects are merely their appearance in conscious awareness. I then introduced the Krauskopf effect, which makes manifest that normal brain processing proceeds by throwing away time- and space-invariant retinal information and inferring it from boundary states. I asserted that this is a true hallucination since what is perceived in the external world is not what is there and that the intermediate causal representation in subsequent brain states is derived from a different part of the external world. I assert that this makes Direct Realism neither necessary nor sufficient for perception. I proposed that a disjunctivist argument is the only escape from this dilemma and made the case that since the Krauskopf effect only makes evident what is a normal neural process, they must thus be disjunctivists about nearly everything we see. I argue that this position is nonfalsifiable.

I then reviewed the remaining Le Morvan counterargument cases to show that each escapes the criticism by weakening what Direct Realism is able to positively assert about perception. I argued that in sum they preclude any prediction from Direct Realism as to what will be seen, preclude invalidation of any logical consequence of the Direct Realism position, and preclude consideration of any contrary experimental evidence, and hence make it nonfalsifiable. I conclude that if all the counterarguments are accepted, Direct Realism has nothing to left to say about perception and that it is defined only by the negative assertion that it is "not indirect."

I believe that many people are supportive of Direct Realism less because they find it a compelling idea in its own right than because they are attracted to epistemological arguments that they believe it supports. In particular, Indirect Realism carries the consequence that our knowledge of the external world must be inferred from the intermediate representations we actually observe rather than the distal objects, whereas it is thought that if the awareness were "direct" and thus not involving any *tertium quid*, our epistemology would be better grounded. Although this seems rather at odds with the concession that our awareness is *causally* indirect, I am relatively agnostic on the epistemology, which I think faces serious difficulties in either case. However, I think it is dangerous to base any argument, epistemological or otherwise, on such a soft foundation as that provided by Direct Realism.

APPENDIX A—A VARIATION ON THE MACH STRIP EXPERIMENT

This version of the Mach Strip experiment illustrates a number of interesting aspects of the interaction between our perceptual system, the brain's motor control system, and our cognitive assumptions about the external world.

How to See It

First fold a sheet of paper across the middle and then fold each half the other direction to make a construction as shown in "A" below. Set it on the floor in front of your chair and view it lengthwise as shown in "B."

The image on your retina is a two-dimensional projection, and so it is ambiguous with respect to the two orientations shown in "B." You now need to make it "stand up" as shown in "C." This requires making a mental shift in your assumptions about its orientation very similar to that required to flip a Necker cube. This can take a bit of practice because your brain knows the real orientation and wants to hold on to it. It will help to close one eye to reduce depth cues and to think of the locations of the upper corners as shown in "C." Some people see it immediately; others need to work on it a bit. After you once see it, it gets easier and with a little practice you can flip it up and down at will (Illustration 4.2).

The next step is to shift your body slowly from right to left and back. You will see the paper shape move, twist, and deform to track your movements.

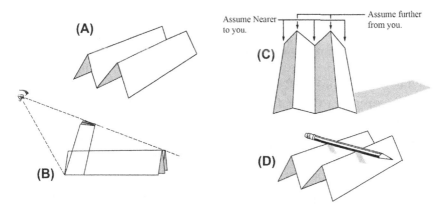

Illustration 4.2 (A) How the paper is folded. (B) How to view it showing actual and illusory positions. (C) How you see it. (D) How the pencil is positioned.

Your brain may reject this and flip it back down again, but with a little practice you can hold it upright while moving freely to and fro and side-to-side. You may also notice other effects as discussed below.

Discussion of the Result

Assuming you now can run the experiment, you no doubt noticed that the object shifted, twisted, and deformed in exactly the required way to both maintain veridical constants such as the alignment of object points with background points, while at the same time honoring your assumption about its three-dimensional orientation. Everything, in fact, remains consistent with the image on the retina.

Depending on your illumination, you might also have noticed that the object appeared to "glow" slightly or have an internal light source in places. This is a similar illusion required to make the assumed three-dimensional orientation consistent with the way the parts of the object shadow itself and produce various luminance values on the retina.

In short, the retinal image, feedback from the motor system, and assumptions about the external world are being kept in registry in real time by what must be an enormous amount of computation that you could not possibly be doing consciously. Indeed, everyone sees the same results whether or not told about them in advance. It is believed that this represents the servoing of an internally maintained best model of the environment to the results of motor action and sensory input. This is a normal process that goes on all the time, but usually the assumptions about the external world are taken from stored learning and prior successful validation of the running model, and so we notice nothing unusual. This is a system that has evolved as a control system for the organism enabling it to operate efficiently on the basis of noisy and incomplete sensory input, and it appears to use exactly the same principles as those of modern control theory (Jagacinski and Flach, 2003).

The system probably did not evolve to serve conscious awareness, and conscious awareness is probably not necessary to its efficient operation, although obviously conscious assumptions may influence the model. The inference usually drawn from the experiment is that it is the servoed internal model, which is presented to our awareness.

As a final demonstration, place a pencil on the paper as shown in "D." This may again cause you difficulty in maintaining the orientation, but a bit of practice will again put you right. I will not spoil it by telling you what you will see, but the answer to "why" is that you are using incorrect assumptions about the paper but not about the pencil.

REFERENCES

Allston, W., 1999. Back to the theory of appearing. Philos. Perspect. 13, 181–203.
Block, M.N., March 2012. An overview of visual hallucinations. Rev. Optom. https://www.reviewofoptometry.com/ce/an-overview-of-hallucinations.
Byrne, A., Logue, H. (Eds.), 2009. Disjunctivism: Contemporary Readings. The MIT Press. ISBN: 978-0-262-02655-0.
Chalmers, D.J., 1996. The Conscious Mind. Oxford University Press.
Collerton, D. (Ed.), December 2014. The Neuroscience of Visual Hallucinations. Wiley-Blackwell. ISBN: 978-1-118-89280-0.
Cotterill, R.M.J., 1996. Prediction and internal feedback in conscious perception. J. Conscious. Stud. 3 (2), 245–266.
Durgin, F.H., Tripathy, S.P., Levi, D.M., 1995. On the filling in the of the visual blind spot. Perception 24, 827–840.
Ewert, J.P., 1985. Concepts in vertebrate neuroethology. Anim. Behav. 33, 1–29.
Flach, J.M., 1990. Control with an eye for perception: precursors to an active psychophysics. Ecol. Psychol. 2 (2), 83–111.
Gordon, G., Kaplan, D.M., Lankow, B., Thaler, L., April 2011. Toward an integrated approach to perception and action: conference report and future directions. Front. Syst. Neurosci. 25.
Hohwy, J., 2012. Attention and conscious perception in the hypothesis testing brain. In: Attention and Consciousness in Different Senses, Frontiers E-books, p. 74.
Horga, G., Schatz, K.C., Abi-Dargham, A., Peterson, B.S., June 11, 2014. Deficits in predictive coding underlie hallucinations in schizophrenia. J. Neurosci. 34 (24), 8072–8082. https://doi.org/10.1523/JNEUROSCI.0200-14.2014.
Huang, Y., Rao, R.P.N., 2011. Predicitve coding. John Wiley & Sons, Ltd. WIREs Cogn. Sci. http://dx.doi.org/10.1002/wcs.142.
Hubel, D.H., Wiesel, T.N., January 1962. Receptive fields, binocular interaction and functional architecture in the cat's visual cortex. J. Physiol. 160 (1), 106–154. http://dx.doi.org/10.1113/jphysiol.

Jagacinski, R.J., Flach, J.M., 2003. Control Theory for Humans: Quantitative Approaches to Modelling Performance. CRC Press.

Kent, E., Albus, J., 1984. Servoed world models as interfaces between robot control systems and sensory data. Robotica 1984 (2), 7–25.

Koenderink, J.J., van Doorn, A.J., 1975. Representation of local geometry in the visual system. Biol. Cybern. 55 (6), 367–375.

Koenderink, J.J., van Doorn, A.J., 1979. The internal representation of solid shape with respect to vision. Biol. Cybern. 32, 211–216.

Komatsu, H., March 2006. The neural mechanisms of perceptual filling-in. Nat. Rev. Neurosci. 7, 220–231.

Komatsu, H., Kinoshita, M., et al., 2000. Neural responses in the retinotopic representation of the blind spot in the macaque V1 to stimuli for perceptual filling-in. J. Neurosci. 20 (24), 9310–9319.

Krauskopof, J., 1963. J. Optom. Soc. Am. 53 (471), 1963.

Le Morvan, P., July 2004. Arguments against direct realism and how to counter them. Am. Philos. Q. 41 (3).

Lizier, J., Prokopenko, M., 2010. Differentiating information transfer and causal effect. Eur. Phys. J. B 73, 605. http://dx.doi.org/10.1140/epjb/e2010-00034-5.

Motoyosh, I., April 1999. Texture filling-in and texture segregation revealed by transient masking. Vis. Res. 39 (7), 285–1291.

Pritchard, R.M., 1962. Stabilized retinal images and visual perception. In: Bernard, E.E., Kare, M.R. (Eds.), Biological Prototypes and Synthetic Systems, Volume 1, Proceedings of the Second Annual Bionics Symposium at Cornell University, Boston, MA. Springer, US, pp. 119–125.

Ramachandran, V.S., Gregory, R.L., April 25, 1991. Perceptual filling in of artificially induced scotomas in human vision. Nature 350, 699–702. http://dx.doi.org/10.1038/350699a0.

Rao, R.P.N., 1999. An optimal estimation approach to visual perception and learning. Vis. Res. 39, 1963–1989.

Sahraiea, A., Hibbardb, P.B., Trevethana, C.T., Ritchiea, K.L., Weiskrantzc, L., 2010. Consciousness of the first order in blindsight. Proc. Natl. Acad. Sci. U.S.A. 107 (49), 21217–21222.

Smythies, J., d'Oreye de Lantremange, M., May 6, 2016. The nature and function of information compression mechanisms in the brain and digital television techniques. Front. Syst. Neurosci. http://dx.doi.org/10.3380/fnsys/2016.00040.

Spillmanna, L., Ottea, T., Hamburgera, K., Magnussenb, S., November 2006. Perceptual filling-in from the edge of the blind spot. Vis. Res. 46 (25), 4252–4257.

Weiskrantz, L., 2007. Blindsight. Scholarpedia 2 (4), 3047.

Wheeler, J., 1989. Information, physics, quantum: the search for links. In: Proc. 3rd Int. Symp. Foundations of Quantum Mechanics, Tokyo, 1989, pp. 354–368.

Wilson, R.A., Keil, F.C. (Eds.), September 1, 2001. The MIT Encyclopedia of the Cognitive Sciences (MITECS) Paperback, p. 311.

Wolpert, D.M., Ghahramani, Z., Jordan, M.I., 1995. An internal model for sensorimotor integration. Science 269 (5232), 1880.

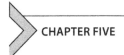

CHAPTER FIVE

Against the Combination of Materialism and Direct Realism

David McGraw

Adjunct Professor, Philosophy, Wayne County Community College, Detroit, MI, United States

In what way—if any—can the duality of physical and phenomenal attributes be avoided? What seems clear is one cannot consistently (1) deny this duality and also (2) affirm conscious experience and also (3) say there is only what is physical. This is what will be argued here.

Some sort of duality seems unavoidable. When Anodos directs his gaze and attention to the wall inside his house, he has the visual impression of the wall. In virtue of having this impression, he apprehends the real wall as a physical thing in the real world of physical things. But this impression is within Anodos and is numerically separate from the wall and its character, functioning, and history. For the wall remains when he closes his eyes and does not see it. The act of apprehending belongs to Anodos and not to the wall. To be sure, the interaction of the wall as a material object with the incoming sunlight, which ultimately results in his visual impression, belongs to the wall. But that is not the same thing as having the visual impression itself belong to the wall.

At least, such a duality seems unavoidable given (1) Anodos lives within a real physical world of real physical things, and (2) the causal functioning of such things impinges on Anodos, and (3) that is why he has the sensory experience. No such duality would exist if objects were mere constructs from experience. In that case, there would in fact not be any physical attributes. More than that, the whole idea of physical attributes would then be out of order. The point of speaking about physical things is to refer to some field or system beyond one's own perceptual impressions, and the concern to do this would be radically misdirected, if objects were mere constructs from experience after all.

There are different ways to develop the thesis that observed objects are mere constructs from experience. The more radical version is phenomenalism, which speaks of such objects as constructed from both actual experiences and hypothetical experiences (which are experiences observers would have if the right conditions were fulfilled). No duality of physical and phenomenal would exist if phenomenalism were true. Only the phenomenal would exist in that case.

The less radical version is what may be called reductive idealism, whereby observed objects are constructed from actual experiences only. But the claim that this version is less radical calls for explanation. Whether reductive idealism is less radical than phenomenalism depends on whether observed objects are claimed to be actually real in some way. If so, then it is less radical. Other things being equal, to construct actual reality from actual elements only is less radical than to construct it from some combination of actual and hypothetical elements.

What if some sort of reductive idealism were true, instead of phenomenalism? Perhaps ordinary observable public objects are wholly constructed from actual experiences, but not necessarily experiences in the minds of human subjects or other higher animals. This might be developed in the manner of Berkeley or whatever. Assuming this would work, what then?

Presumably in that case also, no duality of physical and phenomenal would exist, for there would be nothing physical. To be sure, there might then be some field or system beyond one's own perceptual impressions, as with Berkeley and perhaps some other versions of idealism. But this field or system would not be physical, even though it might be external or objective in some way. An idealist might clam some sort of externality or objectivity for observable things based on his own principles. But even if this claim were to stand up, such things would not be physical. This point comes out clearly in Berkeley's version, in which there are only minds and their ideas. Beyond one's own perceptual impressions, there is God and what he has ordained. But there is nothing (1) of which there are perceptual impressions and (2) that also exists in itself with its own character. With Berkeley, the originals behind the sensory experiences of finite minds are ideas in God's mind only. No other objects of experience exist.

On the other side, assuming that one can speak rightly about physical things, then it would seem there is one's real life within the real world of such things as the basis for sensory experience after all. Given that this is so, what then should be said about the duality of physical and the phenomenal?

Given that the wall is separate from and independent of Anodos's experience in this way, someone might try to avoid the duality by denying the phenomenal side of the division. "Only physical color exists." The claim is there are only the facts of the material world about light and about its reflection and absorption. If what is meant is also that there is no phenomenal color, in the sense that there are not the distinctive qualities of visual experience when one sees red or green or blue, then this claim is clearly false and totally absurd. Human subjects are aware of the colors and other attributes that belong to physical objects as physical only by starting with phenomenal colors and attributes. For one must start from conscious experience of observable objects and their attributes. But what belongs to conscious experience, and thus to such objects and attributes *as consciously presented*, is phenomenal by definition. Apart from experience with its phenomenal character as experience, people would not even have any conception of physical things, let alone any basis for affirming that such things exist.

But what if some radical version of behaviorism or reductive materialism should turn out to be true? What if it should turn out there is no conscious experience? In that case, the duality of physical and phenomenal would be dissolved away, for there would be nothing phenomenal. But by the same token, direct realism would also be false. For there would be nothing phenomenal to be related in any way whatever to the physical, direct, or indirect.

Then again, it seems that phenomenal color is an elaborate construct based on the functioning of the mind and senses. For the phenomenal color within someone's experience can change or cease even apart from any change or cessation of the observed object or in the object's proximate physical environment (leaving aside the body of the observing subject). Thus, one may say phenomenal color does not exist fully and properly since it is less than genuinely real. (The mental event of experiencing is real enough, but the content of this mental event is a mere construct, as being what is developed from the functioning of the mind and senses.) In this sense, only physical color exists. Yes, to be sure, but then the duality of physical and phenomenal is affirmed instead of being avoided. Physical color exists in fact, as belonging to the concrete reality of light and of its reflection and absorption by material things. Phenomenal color exists as a construct within sentient beings.

One might try direct realism (what has been and is called naïve realism). Now, is direct realism true? Are phenomenal attributes a direct reflection of the physical attributes to which they correspond? There are really only so many choices here.

What about simply accepting the phenomenal as something apart from the physical, but as an image of the physical? Could one, on this basis, say rightly that phenomenal attributes are a direct reflection of the physical attributes to which they correspond? Along this line, the denial of the phenomenal may at best be meant, not as a denial of the distinctive character of conscious experience but merely as a sloppy way of answering this question affirmatively. The idea would be there is nothing phenomenal as something different in type or character from the physical. (This point will have to be revisited.)

But no, the phenomenal as an image or direct reflection of the physical will not work, at least not if modern natural science is correct even in its main outlines. For phenomenal attributes differ from physical attributes in type or category and not merely in details. To take obvious examples, the temperature of a volume of water seems to be a simple quality of the water. But in fact, it turns out to be a complicated statistical fact about the vast multitudes of water molecules involved. The tone an object emits seems to be another simple quality, which the object generates. But it turns out to be a cluster of facts about vibration in or by the object and how this vibration affects its environment. The color of an object seems to be yet another simple quality, belonging to the object's surface. But it turns out to be an elaborate cluster of facts about the reflection and absorption of light by that surface, which gets into the complications of quantum physics. Moreover, this concern is not so much about illusions, hallucinations, and other problems that arise. The chief point is: this difference in type or category exists even with veridical perception.

But what does "veridical" mean? One who says material things are fully and properly real means at least that there are things more or less similar or analogous to what is presented to the mind in sensory perception. Naïve versions of realism develop this point by saying veridical perceptual impressions are direct copies of observable facts. But this is not necessary. All that is required is that perceived similarities and differences correspond to similarities and differences that exist as observable facts. For this is enough to make sensory experience conform to real things in an obvious sense of conforming. Veridical impressions may be related to what is objectively real, not so much as a photograph is related to a visible scene but more as a map in an atlas is related to a section of territory, or even as a schematic diagram is related to a circuit.

Furthermore, what is meant by "correspond" in this context can be specified mathematically, in terms of set theory. What is needed is that the perceived relations among things can be rightly mapped into the relations that exist as observable facts. Every experienced similarity and difference (and thus every feature) must line up with some unique similarity or difference (or feature) that exists among the observable facts, and the experience must line up with the fact according to some consistent general rule. But the qualitative richness involved in perception could perfectly well be developed purely within the perceiving subject, even given that the subject's experience is totally veridical, compatibly with sophisticated (but not naïve) realism. Thus, experienced features (within perceptual impressions) must line up with observable features that exist in fact (among external objects) only to the extent of standing in the right (structural) relations to those features that exist in fact. Qualitative matching of experience to fact over and above this, whatever that might mean, is not required for experience to be veridical. For perception can conform to reality even apart from such matching.

What sophisticated realism requires may be brought out by an example. Someone who sees double is not perceiving veridically. This remains true even though both perceived "objects" can be mapped onto some distinct and independent object. For the perceived spatiotemporal separation between the two (apparent) objects cannot be mapped onto anything that exists distinctly from (and independently of) being perceived. More properly, such mapping is not possible based on applying uniformly any consistent general rule for visual experience. (Seeing double is a paradigm case of nonveridical perception exactly because the ability to apply the appropriate rule for visual experience has broken down in such cases.)

Such structural matching is all that is required for experience to be veridical as capturing truly what is there among the things themselves. Compatibly with this kind of correctness, there could be much perceptual processing within the subject, provided this processing does nothing beyond articulating what is already given in some nascent form with the original impressions from the perceived objects. The observed facts whereby such perceptual processing in human subjects involves various weaknesses and limitations are easily accommodated on this basis. Insofar as the structural matching is merely approximate, as being correct only within appropriate tolerances and margins of error, one's experience is less than ideally veridical. Insofar as the processing itself involves faulty interpretations, one is suffering from perceptual tricks and illusions.

Then again, one could try denying that modern natural science is correct, even in its main outlines. But this denial would seem to have disastrous consequences for the underlying concern of exalting the physical as the sole genuine reality. The reason is: modern natural science is largely an outgrowth of the classical realism rooted in ordinary common sense, as being a further development and refinement of such realism. (Classical realism is, roughly, the thesis that sensory experience is based on one's real life within the real world of physical things, where the causal functioning of these things impinges on one's body so as to produce perceptual impressions within oneself.) Therefore, if even the main outlines of this science should fail, then it looks like classical realism would fail along with it. Thus, at worst, this denial might end in reductive idealism, whereby the whole material world is a dream or delusion. Even at best, the basic idea of what it is to be material would have to be reworked. That being so, the whole distinction between mental and material might have to be redrawn.

There is another alternative. Perhaps the phenomenal might be a direct reflection of the physical after all, if neutral monism were true. (Neutral monism is the thesis that both the mental and the material are constructed or developed from something that is "neutral" between the two, as being neither, or perhaps both, or perhaps even both and neither.)

However, even if neutral monism would work, it might not save the original concern that motivates people to deny the duality. Someone might deny the duality to say there is only what is physical or material. But of course, one who affirms neutral monism cannot say this, for what is physical or material will not be primary. It will be just as much of a construct as mind or consciousness, and mind will have just as much basis to be genuinely real as what is material.

To be sure, given neutral monism, it will be false that mind or consciousness is primary or even fully autonomous. Now, in some cases, the concern to deny both the primacy and the autonomy of the mental may in fact be the underlying motivation. What value this denial has given neutral monism will then depend on what the underlying reality of both the mental and the material turns out to be. This point will have to be revisited.

Finally, one might try panpsychism. (Panpsychism is, roughly, the thesis that all things—even subatomic particles—have some sort of mental activity or character belonging to their essential nature.) But once again, even if that would work, the underlying concern would be lost. For then ordinary observable public objects would be radically different from what has been traditionally understood in the West. To affirm panpsychism is to say material bodies, simply and strictly as such, have some sort of mental life going on inside them. But then they are living beings. This is contrary to the traditional basic assumption that material things as such, insofar as they are material and apart from being organized into appropriate structures, are passively responsive, merely receptive and reactive, with nothing like their own agency or autonomy. Given all this, the whole distinction between mental and material would have to be redrawn.

In fact, what panpsychism involves is even more serious than that. Properly speaking, panpsychism could be considered a form of idealism. For if panpsychism were true, then it would be true that nothing nonmental exists. Yet this is not a form of reductive idealism, unlike what Berkeley had. For even with panpsychism, things such as shape, size, position, and velocity would still be genuinely real, instead of being mere constructs from experiences. But what then?

The answer depends on what the basis is for material bodies to be what they are and do what they do. These material attributes would be genuinely real, but they would be developed out of the being's inner functioning somehow. Since this inner functioning is its mental life, these things would be developed out of the being's inner functioning as something mental. In that case, observable objects would still be material, as opposed to being purely spiritual in the manner of an angel or of God. But even if nothing existed other than beings that are material in this way, classical materialism would still be false, for the dominant basis for things would be mental life instead of material attributes and functions.

However, since the basic distinction between mental and material is one of the chief concerns at issue here, what it means to say the "basis for things would be mental life instead of material attributes and functions" is problematic, not clear or obvious. The best answer seems to be to see what is distinctive about the mental that is relevant here and how this contrasts with the material.

Mental activity is largely concerned with shaping means to ends. This concern is so important that James took it to be the defining attribute of mind.[1] It is at least one of the central features of mental life. On the other side, the lack or absence of concern with ends and goals seems to be one of the distinctive or even defining features of material things insofar as they are material and of things that work in some purely material way. A material device, simply and strictly as such, is void of all ability to look to the rationale of any process as a whole and act on that basis.

On this basis, one may speak of a being's mental life as that being's system of desires and purposes, and also of the feelings and awareness (including memories and thoughts as well as perceptual impressions) strongly associated with those desires and purposes. By contrast, insofar as something is

[1] James, 1950. 1:6–11.

merely material, there is the concrete reality of whatever attributes (both monadic and relational) it happens to embody—most obviously geometric attributes—and that is all the thing is, as well as whole the basis for it to do what it does. There is no concern with ends or goals, and nothing like the feelings or awareness strongly associated with such concern.

Therefore, to say the basis for things would be mental life instead of material attributes and functions if panpsychism were true means things such as shape, size, position, velocity, and so on would *not* be just the concrete reality of what is embodied and what happens on that basis, and that is all. Nor would these things be only the outgrowth or implementation of something further that happens to be embodied in concrete reality, and that is all. Instead, this whole structure of what is merely embodied in concrete reality would somehow manifest the being's interior processes of feelings, desires, awareness, and so on. Moreover, these interior processes (or at least the most basic of them) would not be themselves reducible to what is nonmental. Of course, if all this were so, materialism as traditionally understood would be false.

In one way, the problem of qualia can be left aside here. This is so even though this problem is often considered one of the great difficulties about reducing mind to body. For all that has been said so far, a material being's attributes and processes could perhaps involve plenty of qualitative richness and vividness, and yet the being might still be totally nonmental. This will be so, provided such richness and vividness are merely embodied in concrete reality as belonging to what the thing is, apart from any basis of feeling, desire, or awareness.

The question about an observable object's character and behavior can also be developed in another way. This approach will show even more directly the failure of materialism and naïve realism to mix.

Given naïve or direct realism, the claim is, the phenomenal attributes to be found in people's experience are a direct reflection of the real physical character of the real physical object. In that case, such attributes belong to the object as being what the object is in itself. But then, what the object displays is these attributes as they are to be found in conscious awareness. For that is what "direct reflection" means in this context.

Such phenomenal features will also be the operational attributes of the object. The exercise of these attributes will be the basis for things to work as they do. So, for example, hot water will dissolve things better than cold water, not because of complicated facts down at the molecular level but because the simple quality of heat is more powerful than the simple quality of cold. This is what shows up at the phenomenal level, and what is real is directly reflected on that level. Again, photochemistry will work, not because of quantum physics but because of the interplay of the qualities involved, *as qualities*. In general, the interplay of observable attributes as such will be the basis for the behavior as well as the character of things.

Thus, the basis for things will be phenomenal attributes. But these attributes are just that—phenomenal. Therefore, at best neutral monism will be true. Moreover, even though one can still rightly deny both the primacy and the autonomy of the mental, yet the nature of reality will turn out to have such a heavy slant toward mind or consciousness that the result will be at least seriously repugnant to the main thrust of classical materialism. At worst, the basis will be some sort of mental life, even if material attributes and functions are also real. But then, even if full panpsychism can be avoided, the underlying concerns of classical materialism will be lost.

Yet there may seem to be some basis for question here, in spite of all these points. For there can be an enormous temptation to accept naïve or direct realism. But, for one who favors materialism on other grounds, the denial of materialism may seem to be an exorbitant price to pay for such acceptance. The line of least resistance might then be to try to combine both.

In the present context, whether materialism should be accepted on its own merits can be left aside as a debate for another day. However, the temptation to accept naïve or direct realism can be shown to be just that—a temptation. There are critical distinctions that must be drawn.

Assuming there is the duality of physical and phenomenal attributes, what does this fact involve, or how does it work? The color of the wall Anodos sees is a physical feature of the wall and belongs to the concrete reality of the physical world. But the awareness Anodos has of that color is phenomenal and is within Anodos as resulting from his functioning as a sentient being. "Does this mean he does not see the wall as it truly is?" No, for here is the first distinction that must be drawn. Locke said people think of perceivable attributes as being perceived by the senses the way objects are reflected in a mirror.[2] But this is not necessary, as Locke himself understood. To perceive something truly, it is enough that someone's experience be veridical, in the sense of "veridical" that has been set forth here. On this basis, Anodos may be seeing the wall as it is, even though the phenomenal quality in his experience differs in character from the physical color of the wall.

---

[2] Locke, 1975. 2.8.16.

"Then, does he fail to perceive the wall directly?" No, for here is the second distinction that must be drawn. To be sure, Anodos does not "directly apprehend" the wall or any other real physical thing as having such things in direct and immediate contact with his soul, so to speak (which, in this context, is to say—with the inner life of one's character and capabilities as an intellectual being). That is not how experience based on perceiving through the senses works. But the elaborate processes that occur within Anodos when he sees or hears or touches, which modern science has partially uncovered, are not things that happen instead of, or as obstructions to, sensory perception. The appropriate biological processes *are* the processes of perceiving through the senses. To go through such processes is to perceive through the senses. The correct question is only whether or how far some distortion has or has not been introduced by these processes. Thus, one who follows modern natural science can affirm classical realism by saying sensory experience is caused by interactions among material things and also corresponds to facts that are present among such things, at least in the sense of formal mapping. Indeed, such experience lines up with what is material exactly because it is derived from what is material. In this way, modern science allows for the real relations of experienced objects to perceiving subjects, as well as the objects themselves, to be apprehended rightly. Classical realism is vindicated on this basis.

This way of being related to objects seems to be exactly what happens whenever anyone sees or touches any object.[3] Unhappily, though, Locke tried to affirm that sensory experience backs up classical realism, but he spoke sometimes as though "ideas" in the mind were what is really perceived.[4] But what is needed (and what is proposed here) is rather the old Aristotelian idea that the things themselves are perceived by means of various sensory faculties and mental structures.[5] Given that people perceive their own sensations (instead of perceiving objects by means of sensations), there will not be the required relations of the perceiving subject to the things themselves. For then the relations involved in perceiving will reach from the subject only to the sensations rather than to the (external) things. So, if this were the way sensory perception works, then one would not be able to affirm classical realism.

However, the thesis that impressions rather than objects are perceived is really not plausible. Sensory experiences are clearly not perceived in

[3] Locke, 1975. 2.9.1–4, 4.2.14, 4.4.1–4, 4.11.1–7, 4.13.2.
[4] Locke, 1975. 2.1.1, 2.2.1, 2.8.8, 4.1.1, 4.2.14, 4.17.8.
[5] Aristotle, 350 BC. 2.5, 2.12.424a16–24, 3.2.425b11–426b7.

anything like the way objects appear to be perceived. For example, when someone sees a rock, he does not need to look at a visual impression of the rock as he might look at a (material) painting or photograph. He does not even need to introspect and examine it as he might examine an image from a dream. Instead, the whole awareness of the (external) object is the sensory experience that is supposedly perceived. To have that kind of impression in that way is already to see the rock. Nothing more is required.

The argument proposed here is essentially similar to Moore's argument concerning the nature of sensation. Sensory awareness seems to be "transparent" or "diaphanous." An experience points to its object and not to itself as a mental act.[6]

Given that perception does involve apprehending real relations of observable things to oneself, then real things are what stand "at the other end" of veridical perception. According to classical realism, real things are present to perceiving subjects in exactly this way. The awareness of real things is as direct as possible for beings who perceive through the senses, instead of apprehending directly through immediate contact of the known object with the soul (which, in this context, is to say—with the inner life of one's character and capabilities as an intellectual being).

Thus, when Anodos sees the wall, there is the visual impression of the wall within him, and to have that impression is already to perceive the real wall in the real world. But the wall itself, as it exists in itself, is and remains external to Anodos, as do all its parts (including surfaces), and all its individual attributes. What is within Anodos is only an effect of some appropriate process involving the wall. He does not partake of the wall itself. The observed duality of physical and phenomenal results from these facts and so is not to be denied.

Yet, exactly because sensory experience is transparent or diaphanous, it may still seem one can deny (the existence of) phenomenal attributes as separate from physical attributes, although in another way. As Tye points out, there is the experience of the object with its attributes, and there is the introspective awareness of this experience, and that is all. There are no phenomenal attributes other than the attributes of observable things as presented in experience.[7]

Yes, indeed so. But it does not follow that phenomenal features and attributes are a direct reflection of the physical, let alone that phenomenal features and attributes are numerically identical with those of observed

[6] Moore, 1922. 17–27.
[7] Tye, 2002. 51–54.

physical things. For the manner in which observable attributes are presented in consciousness is a function of the perceiving subject. The tricks and illusions to which the senses are subject illustrate this point very clearly, and these tricks and illusions are important in this context chiefly for that reason. But the principle applies generally and holds good even with experience that is veridical in the sense explained here. What is developed within the subject depends on how the subject happens to be affected. But this effect on the subject is an external accident from the standpoint of the perceived object. (e.g., the fact that people find sucrose and sodium chloride to have the distinctive tastes they have is much less a fact about those chemicals and much more a fact about human subjects. What people taste is an external accident from the standpoint of the chemicals.) Even at best, there is no guarantee that what arises in the mind of the subject will be at all a direct reflection of what the perceived object is within itself, from its own standpoint. Indeed, experience shows the truth to be the opposite. Given modern natural science, the way in which the phenomenal portrays the physical will not support both direct realism and materialism.

FURTHER READING

Aristotle, 350 BC, On the Soul.
James, W., 1890. The Principles of Psychology. Henry Holt & Co., n.p., Reprint, Dover Publications, New York, 1950.
Locke, J., 1975. In: Nidditch, P.H. (Ed.), An Essay Concerning Human Understanding. Clarendon Press, Oxford, London, n.p., 1690.
Moore, G.E., 1922. The refutation of idealism (Chapter). In: Ogden, C.K. (Ed.), Philosophical Studies. International Library of Psychology, Philosophy, and Scientific Method Kegan Paul, Trench, Trubner & Co., Ltd., London, 1922; Harcourt, Brace and Company, New York.
Tye, M., 2000. Consciousness, Color, and Content. Representation and Mind Series. MIT Press, Cambridge, MA. MIT Press Paperback Edition, 2002.

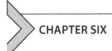

CHAPTER SIX

The Epistemology of Visual Experience

Steven Lehar
Independent Researcher, Manchester, MA, United States

1. THE EPISTEMOLOGICAL DIVIDE

The scientific investigation into the nature of biological vision has been plagued by a persistent confusion over the question whether the world we see around us in visual consciousness is the real world itself or whether it is merely a perceptual replica of that world in an internal representation. In other words this is the question of *Direct Perception* as opposed to *Indirect Perception*. Direct perception, also known as *Direct Realism*, or *Naïve Realism*, is the natural intuitive understanding of vision that we accept without question from the earliest days of childhood, i.e., that the world we see around us is the world itself. Indirect Perception, also known as *Indirect Realism*, or *Representationalism* suggests on the other hand that the world we see around us is not the real world itself but merely a perceptual replica of that world in an internal representation (Smythies, 1989, 1994).

The distinction between these two views of perception is illustrated schematically in Fig. 6.1. In the direct realist view, your perceptual experience of the world around you as you sit reading this book is identified as the world itself, i.e., you perceive yourself where you sit, surrounded by your physical environment, as suggested in Fig. 6.1A. In the indirect realist view of perception, the world you see around you is identified as a miniature perceptual copy of the world contained within your real physical head, as suggested schematically in Fig. 6.1B. The external world and your true physical head are depicted in dashed lines, to indicate that these entities are invisible to your direct experience.

A number of intermediate alternatives have been proposed over the years, whereby experience is indeed a product of the physical brain, but that experience is not itself located in the brain, it is either projected out of the brain to appear superimposed on the external world, as it appears to naïve perception (Velmans, 1990), or that experience has no spatial location either in the brain or outside of it (Dennett, 1991; Pessoa et al., 1998;

Direct versus Indirect Realism
ISBN 978-0-12-812141-2
https://doi.org/10.1016/B978-0-12-812141-2.00006-4

73

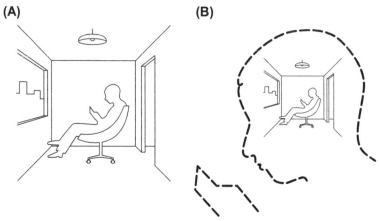

Figure 6.1 (A) Your perceptual experience of the world as you sit reading this book, as conceptualized in the direct view of perception. (B) The true situation as conceived in the philosophy of indirect perception, where your percept of the world around you is identified as an internal pattern in your head, the real external world (shown in dashed lines) being beyond your direct experience.

Gibson, 1972). These theories suggest that experience is a subjective non-physical entity that is in principle undetectable by physical means. Some even suggest that visual consciousness does not exist as we experience it but is actually a lot more impoverished than we experience it to be (Dennett, 1991, 1992).

The reason for the continued confusion on this issue is that all three alternatives are frankly incredible. Direct Perception is incredible because it suggests that we can have experience out beyond the sensory surface, in violation of everything we know about the causal chain of vision. The phenomena of dreams and hallucinations are problematic for Direct Perception because they demonstrate the capacity of the brain to construct complete virtual worlds, a capacity which must surely be employed also in normal spatial perception, as revealed by many visual illusions. Furthermore, Direct Perception offers no clue as to how an artificial vision system could possibly be endowed with the kind of external perception that we observe in visual consciousness. The theory of Direct Perception is as mysterious as the property of consciousness, which it attempts to explain.

Indirect Perception is also incredible, for it suggests that the world that we see around us is actually inside our head. This can only mean that the head, which we have come to know as our own is not our true physical head, but merely a miniature perceptual copy of our head inside a perceptual replica of the world, all of which is contained within our physical head. Indirect Perception suggests a three-dimensional volumetric imaging mechanism in the brain for which no direct neurophysiological evidence has been found.

Projection theory is also incredible because its explanation of the spatial structure of experience is that it is a purely subjective structure that has no mass, occupies no space, consumes no energy, and is undetectable in principle in the physical world known to science. This makes projection theory an *unfalsifiable* hypothesis because its prediction, that experience will not be detected, is identical to the *null* prediction that nothing is projected. It is as if the solid spatial structure of the world that we experience around us had no existence in the physical world, and is thus not a valid subject for scientific scrutiny; something to be ignored, or explained away as a pseudoproblem, as if the magnificent edifice of visual consciousness were of no consequence to science. But this is a curious inversion of the true epistemology whereby the sense data of experience are the *only thing* that we can be certain to actually exist. Our knowledge of our own experience is primary, unmediated. It is as it appears to be. All else, including the entire world of science, is an elaborate inference based on that experience.

As for the *eliminative hypothesis*, the argument that visual consciousness can be "explained" by denying its existence as a spatial image (Dennett, 1991), this is a straight contradiction in terms. I can be absolutely certain when I am having an experience that has the properties that I experience it to have. To claim otherwise is to fly in the face of the very definition of experience. More importantly, to deny the scientific significance of this most compelling of all illusions is to ignore the most interesting and challenging part of the problem of vision as if it *did not exist*. A neuroscience that explains everything about visual processing except for the experience of visual consciousness is a neuroscience that explains essentially *nothing* because it is visual consciousness that makes the visual brain interesting in the first place.

2. A HISTORY OF THE EPISTEMIC DEBATE

The question of the epistemology of conscious experience has a long and colorful history in psychology and philosophy. The epistemological question is intimately related to the issue of mind–body dualism because all of the problems inherent in the naïve realist view simply evaporate if we allow for the existence of an immaterial soul, whose function is not entirely dependent on the mechanical functioning of the physical brain.

For in visual perception we do indeed feel as if our consciousness extends outward beyond the confines of our physical head, to make direct sensory contact with remote objects in the world. But while the external nature of perception has been recognized into ancient times, so too has the causal role of the sensory organs in perception, for the world goes dark when we close our eyes and disappears altogether when we lose our eyes. We have therefore two fundamental and apparently contradictory observations on the nature of vision, one that appears to lead inward from the world through the eye to the brain as revealed by physiology, while the other appears to lead outward from the mind to the external visual world as revealed by phenomenology. With the rise of the materialistic world view ushered in by Newton's mechanical universe, there has been ever increasing pressure to formulate a materialistic explanation for the mystery of visual consciousness.

As we review the history of this issue, a gradual progression is observed, as ever more of the properties of the phenomenal world, initially assumed to be identical to the external world, is attributed instead to processes internal to the mind and brain. This leaves the phenomenal portions of the external world in a peculiar kind of limbo, being observed external to the body while being attributed to processes within the body. The ultimate solution to this paradox is only to be found by a complete indirect realist inversion, whereby everything that appears to be external is finally attributed unambiguously to internal processes in the brain, a view, which forever closes the naïve window of direct observation onto the external world.

The first stage of the epistemological inversion was proposed by Descartes, who as an anatomist, observed that the optic nerve connected the eye to the brain. Since Kepler had already demonstrated that the lens of the eye projects an image on the retina, Descartes proposed that the optic nerve sends the image from the retina up to the brain where it is "seen" by the immaterial "soul," which he supposed to connect to the brain at the pineal gland (Pastore, 1971, p. 19). This, however, leaves the "seeing" part of the problem to an immaterial soul that is in principle beyond scientific scrutiny. This theory, which is related to projection theory, is similarly unfalsifiable. However, as flawed as this explanation may be as a scientific hypothesis, it does have the distinct merit of corresponding closely to our subjective experience whereby we open our eyes to the world and see the world "out there" beyond our retinal surface.

John Locke took the next step of the epistemological inversion by proposing that we cannot see the world directly at all, what we see is the product of the image on our retina sent up the optic nerve, processed and interpreted by our brain. However, Locke retained a residual aspect of direct perception in his distinction between the *primary* and *secondary* qualities of perception. The primary qualities, which include shape, size, and number, are, he claimed, a veridical representation of the actual properties of the objects themselves, while the secondary qualities such as color, smell, and taste are also produced by stimulation of sense, but they have no resemblance to the corresponding qualities in the objects (Pastore, 1971, p. 64–66). The isolation of the soul from direct contact with the external world led Bishop Berkeley to question the very existence of the external world, for since we cannot see it directly, how can we know that it even exists? Berkeley therefore professed a form of idealism, whereby mind is all that really exists, as captured by Berkeley's dictum that "to be is to be perceived." As long as the choice is restricted to epistemological monist alternatives, the choice is between two incredible possibilities, either naïve realism or idealism.

Immanuel Kant completed the epistemological inversion by proposing that there are two worlds of reality: The *noumenal* world, i.e., the objective external world known to science, and the *phenomenal* world, which is the subjective world of our experience. Kant explained that these are separate and distinct worlds, but only one of them, the phenomenal world, is manifest to our direct experience. All we can ever know of the noumenal world is by its effects on the phenomenal world. However, Kant's epistemology was somewhat confused by his belief that the noumenal world was not a physical world but was also a world of mind, although it was the mind of God, an objective external mind that contains all of our individual minds. And minds contain "ideas," which in the usage of the time included mental and sensory images, and thus the noumenal and phenomenal worlds both contained images such as those in our visual experience, dreams, and hallucinations. The problem of vision became more challenging after the French Materialist philosophers finally banished Gods and spirits from our scientific explanations of the world and proposed that animals are biological automata, no different in principle from artificial robots.

The critical realist philosophers (Sellars, 1916; Russell, 1921; Broad, 1925; Drake, 1920) named the vivid spatial structure of visual experience as the "sense data" of experience, thus highlighting the fact that the spatially extendedness of experience was an extendedness of the experience itself, not only of the external object that it represents. In other words, shape and location are secondary qualities also, in Locke's sense, i.e., there is no aspect of perception, which is a primary manifestation of the external world. The idea of sense data suggests that visual experience is like a museum diorama, or a theater set, painted in bright colors to look just like the scene it represents. This identification of sense data as belonging unambiguously to subjective experience raises the question of where this spatial structure could possibly be located, and the critical realists were divided on whether sense data were located in the brain or out in the world, or whether they were purely subjective and thus located in no particular place.

Bertrand Russell, originally himself a critical realist, eventually discovered the resolution to this quandary with a realist version of Kant's epistemological dualism. What finally convinced Russell was consideration of the *causal chain of vision*. Light from an object in the world enters the eye, where it is transduced to a neural signal on the retina, sent up the optic nerve, from whence it is eventually transformed into a pattern of activation in the brain that causes an experience of the object. If that activation is located in your brain, then the experience that it generates must also be located in your brain. To claim that experience is something different than the patterns of activation in the brain is to invoke a dualism whereby experience is something other than the physical operation of the physical brain. The Gestalt movement, especially Kurt Koffka (1935), Wolfgang Köhler and Held (1947), and Wolfgang Köhler (1971), reached the same epistemological conclusion independently and argued eloquently for the representational nature of perception. Gestalt visual illusions reveal the capacity of the brain to construct illusory spatial structures in perception, a constructive image-like capacity as seen also in dreams and hallucinations.

Russell (1927, p. 137–143) observed that a potent source of confusion in this matter is a confusion of physical space with perceptual space. For although our percept of the external world appears external to our head, it is not external to our true physical head but only to our perceptual head in perceptual space. All of our perceptual space, including the externally perceived world, is inside our physical head in physical space (Russell, 1927). This explanation of perception finally resolved all of the epistemological problems inherent in naïve realism and in idealism without resort to any supernatural gods or mystical souls. It accounts for the fact that the perceived world appears external although we know it to be internal, by the fact that the external world of perception is internal to our physical brain. It accounts for the realism known to common sense, by the fact that the phenomenal world, while truly internal and shut-in within the physical brain, nevertheless accurately reflects certain geometrical aspects of the external world, which is thereby knowable indirectly through its perceptual replica. It accounts for the fact that different individuals each have their own unique perspective on a commonly viewed object by the fact that each individual percipient has his/her own private perceptual copy of that object. Bertrand Russell's epistemological dualism and causal theory of perception should therefore have *resolved the epistemological question once and for all*. But curiously it did not. And the reason why it has failed to do so is almost as interesting and significant as the epistemological question itself.

The epistemological debate highlights the very powerful human inclination to favor a naïve realist view. After all we are all born naïve realists, and only a few in each generation ever come to see through the grand illusion of conscious experience. Russell's causal theory of perception has never been refuted, and yet it continues to be simply ignored or misunderstood, although each of the alternatives has been repeatedly shown to be fatally flawed. The chief problem is that indirect realism seems so incredible on the face of it that it is most often not even considered as a serious alternative.

3. THE WORLD IN YOUR HEAD

One reason for the persistent confusion over the epistemological question is that Russell's insight is particularly difficult to visualize or to explain in unambiguous terms. For example, even the description of the causal chain of vision is itself somewhat ambiguous since it can be interpreted in two alternative ways. Consider the statement that light from this page stimulates an image in your eye, which in turn promotes the formation of a percept of the page up in your brain. The ambiguity inherent in this statement can be revealed by the question "where is the percept?" There are two alternative correct answers to this question, although each is correct in a different spatial context. One answer is that the percept is up in your head, (the one you point to when asked to point to your head) which is correct in the external or direct realist context of your perceived head being identified with your objective physical head, and since your visual cortex is contained within your head that must also be the location of the patterns of energy corresponding to your percept of the page. The problem with this answer, however, is that no percept is experienced within your head where you imagine your visual cortex to be located. The other correct answer is that the percept of the page is right here in front of you where you experience the image of a page. This answer is correct in the internal spatial context of the entire perceived world around you being within your head. However, the problem with this answer is that there is now no evidence of the objective external page that serves as the source of the light. The problem is that the vivid spatial structure you see before you is serving two mutually inconsistent roles, both as a mental icon representing the objective external page, which is the original source of the light, and as an icon of the final percept of the page inside your head; i.e., the page you see before you represents both ends of the causal chain. And our mental image of the problem switches effortlessly between the internal and external contexts to focus on each end of the causal chain in turn. It is this automatic switching of mental context that makes this issue so elusive because it hinders a consideration of the problem as a whole.

I propose an alternative mental image to disambiguate the two spatial contexts that are so easily confused (Lehar, 2003a,b). I propose that out beyond the farthest things you can perceive in all directions, i.e., above the dome of the sky and below the solid earth under your feet, or beyond the walls, floor, and ceiling of the room you see around you, are located the inner surface of your true physical skull. And beyond that skull is an unimaginably immense external world of which the world you see around you is merely a miniature internal replica. In other words, the head you have come to know as your own is not your true physical head, but only a miniature perceptual copy of your head in a perceptual copy of the world, all of which is contained within your real head in the external objective world. This mental image is more than just a metaphorical device, for the perceived and objective worlds are not spatially superimposed, as is assumed in the direct realist model, but the perceived world is completely contained within your head in the objective world. Although this statement can only be true in a topological, rather than a strictly topographical sense, the advantage of this mental image is that it provides two separate and distinct icons for the separate and distinct internal and external worlds that can now coexist within the same mental image. This no longer allows the automatic switching between spatial contexts that tends to confuse the issue. Furthermore, this insight emphasizes the indisputable fact that every aspect of the solid spatial world that we perceive to surround us is in fact primarily a manifestation of activity within an internal representation, and only in secondary fashion is it also representative of more distant objects and events in the external world (Fig. 6.2).

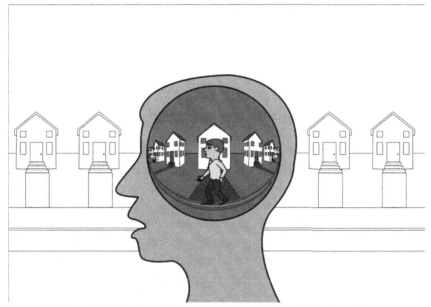

Figure 6.2 Beyond the farthest things you can perceive in all directions, is your true physical skull, and beyond that skull is an unimaginably immense external world of which the world you see around you is a miniature internal replica.

I have found a curious dichotomy in the response of colleagues in discussions on this issue. For when I say that everything you perceive is inside your head, they are apt to reply "why of course, but that is so obvious it need hardly be stated." When on the other hand I turn that statement around and say that their physical skull is located out beyond the farthest things they can perceive around them, to this they object "Impossible! You must be mad!" And yet the two statements are logically identical! How can it be that the one is blindingly obvious, while the other seems patently absurd? This provocative formulation of the issue in the double mental image is my contribution to the debate, for it brings into sharper focus a concept that is difficult to address in more abstracted terms.

4. THE GEOMETRY OF VISUAL SPACE

The most persuasive evidence for the indirectness of perception can be seen in the geometry of visual space (Lehar, 2003a,b). If you stand on a long straight road or railway track the sides of the road appear to converge to a vanishing point where they apparently meet, and if you turn around and look behind you, they converge to a point behind also. Topologically speaking therefore the road is shaped like the rind of a melon slice with sides that meet at a point at each end, and yet those sides appear straight and parallel and equidistant throughout their length. Fig. 6.3A shows the perceptual experience of a man on a long straight road. Fig. 6.3B shows the same scene overlaid with an infinite Euclidean grid warped by the same perspective projection as that of visual experience. The curved lines represent a grid of parallel straight lines.

Perhaps the most curious feature of this warped geometry is that it is practically invisible to most people until it is pointed out to them. And even then, some deny vociferously that they perceive any perspective foreshortening at all with distance. For example, Eric Schwitzgebel (2006) argues adamantly that he does not see the sides of the road converging to a vanishing point in *any sense*. He sees the sides of the road as perfectly straight and parallel and equidistant all the way up to where they appear to meet on the horizon.

Do the sides of the road appear to converge? Or are they perceived to be straight and parallel throughout their length? Does the far end of a hallway appear smaller by perspective, or does the hallway appear perfectly parallel and rectangular? Do objects in the distance appear smaller by perspective, or do they appear undiminished in size? It took me months of the most intense introspective observation before I could answer this question to my own satisfaction. Standing in a hallway, sometimes I would decide that the walls appear to converge, other times I saw them as perfectly parallel. It seemed to switch with my mood, or mental set, and I really

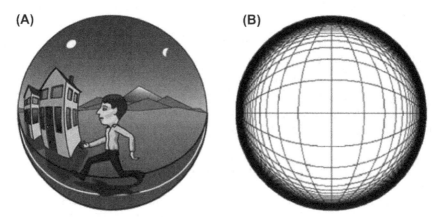

Figure 6.3 (A) The perceptual experience of a man on a long straight road. (B) The perspective projection of that experience, representing an infinite grid of parallel straight lines.

could not decide between them. I finally discovered the solution to this apparent paradox with the answer of *both!* Objects in the distance appear smaller by perspective, and yet at the same time they also appear undiminished in size. It is the size scale of phenomenal space that shrinks with distance, such that shrunken objects in the distance are measured against a shrunken metric scale and are thus perceived undiminished in size. If the grid lines of Fig. 6.3B are used to judge the straightness of the lines in the experience in Fig. 6.3A, you will see that the sides of the road are straight and parallel and equidistant throughout their length. In Fig. 6.3A the two houses appear to be of different size, but they span the same number of grid lines in Fig. 6.3B and are thus perceived to be of the same objective size. The farther house is merely presented at lower perceptual resolution, it is both smaller, and not smaller all at the same time.

I conducted an experiment in a hallway at the Schepens Eye Research Institute (Lehar, 1999) to demonstrate phenomenal perspective. Subjects placed in the hallway were given three cardboard models, as shown in Fig. 6.4A and asked to choose which model most closely resembled their experience of the surrounding hallway: Not the shape that they "knew" it to have, but the shape that they experienced the hallway to have. Did it appear like a rectangular prism, like model A? Or did it look like a flat two-dimensional perspective projection as in model C? Or did the hallway appear intermediate, a kind of bas-relief shape as in model B? Subjects' responses were split about evenly between models A and B. Then the subjects were given a fourth model D, depicted in Fig. 6.4B, which was identical to the bas-relief model B except this time etched with grid lines. The subjects were told that the grid lines represent the scale of the model, and that scale varied with depth, such that objects in the distance were presented at a smaller scale as compared with objects in the foreground, as indicated by the converging grid lines. When offered this alternative, all the subjects chose this one because *this model embodies the same duality in size perception observed in phenomenal perspective*, whereby objects in the distance are perceived to be smaller by perspective, and yet at the same time they are perceived to be undiminished in size.

Perspective is traditionally defined as a projection from a three-dimensional world onto a two-dimensional surface, such as the retina, or the film plane of a camera. But the world of experience is not a flat two-dimensional projection; it is a solid volumetric world that exhibits a perspective distortion. Nowhere in the objective world of external reality is there anything remotely resembling perspective as we observe it in phenomenal experience.

(A)   **(B)**

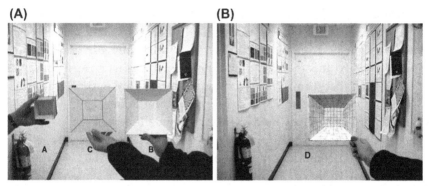

Figure 6.4 (A) The "Hallway Experiment:" in which subjects are asked to select which of three cardboard models most closely resembles their experience of the surrounding hallway. (B) A fourth cardboard model etched with grid lines that represent the shrinking spatial scale due to perspective.

The prominent violation of Euclidean geometry evident in phenomenal perspective is perhaps the clearest evidence for the world of experience as an internal rather than an external entity, for the curvature of perceived space is clearly not a property of the world itself, only of our perceptual representation of it. What does it mean for a space to be curved? If it is the space itself, which is curved, rather than just the objects within that space, then it is the definition of straightness itself, which is curved in that space. In other words if the space were filled with a set of grid lines marking straight lines with uniform spacing, as shown in Fig. 6.3B, those lines themselves would be curved rather than straight, as they are in Euclidean space. However, the curvature would not be apparent to creatures that live in that curved space because the curves that are followed by those grid lines are the very definition of straightness in that space. In other words a curved object in that curved space would be defined as perfectly straight, as long as the curvature of the object exactly matched the curvature of the space it was in. If you are having difficulty picturing this paradoxical concept and suspect that it embodies a contradiction in terms, just look at phenomenal perspective, which has exactly that paradoxical property. For phenomenal perspective embodies exactly that same contradiction in terms, with parallel lines meeting at two points while passing to either side of the percipient and while being perceived to be straight and parallel and equidistant throughout their length. This absurd contradiction is clearly not a property of the physical world, which is measurably Euclidean at least at the familiar scale of our everyday environment. Therefore that curvature must be a property of perceived space, thereby confirming that perceived space is not the same as the external space of which it is an imperfect replica.

In fact, the observed warping of perceived space is exactly the property that allows a finite representational space to encode an infinite external space. This property is achieved by using a variable representational scale, i.e., the ratio of the physical distance in the perceptual representation relative to the distance in external space that it represents. This scale is observed to vary as a function of distance from the center of our perceived world, such that objects close to the body are encoded at a larger representational scale than objects in the distance, and beyond a certain limiting distance the representational scale, at least in the depth dimension, falls to zero, i.e., objects beyond a certain distance lose all further perceptual depth. This is seen, for example, where the sun and moon and distant mountains appear as if cut out of paper and pasted against the dome of the sky.

5. ANALOGICAL REPRESENTATION AND INFORMATION THEORY

Once we recognize the world of experience for what it really is, it becomes clearly evident that the representational strategy used by the brain is an *analogical* one (Lehar, 2003a, 2003b). In other words, objects and surfaces are represented in the brain neither by an abstract symbolic code, as suggested in the propositional paradigm nor are they encoded by the activation of individual cells or groups of cells representing particular features detected in the scene, as suggested in the neural network or feature detection paradigm. Instead, objects are represented in the brain by constructing full spatial effigies of them that appear to us for all the world like the objects themselves—or at least so it seems to us only because we have never seen those objects in their raw form but only through our perceptual representations of them. Indeed the only reason why this very obvious fact of perception has been so often overlooked is because the illusion is so compelling that we tend to mistake the world of perception for the real world of which it is merely a copy. This is a classic case of not seeing the forest for the trees, for the evidence for the nature of perceptual representation in the brain has been right before us all along, cleverly disguised as objects and surfaces in a virtual world that we take to be reality. It is, however, apparently the ultimate paradigm shift, one that requires one to turn one's mental reality totally inside-out, a mental inversion not everybody is willing to make.

(A)   **(B)**

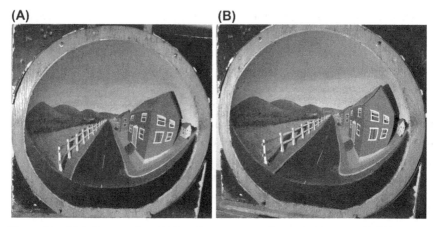

Figure 6.5 (A) A diorama that depicts the curvature of perceived space. (B) Oblique view.

Fig. 6.5 shows a diorama that I built to depict the curvature of perceived space as I perceive it in my experience. If the photograph in Fig. 6.5A had been taken from the "egocentric point," or center of the perceptual sphere, the curved sides of the road and the fence line would appear perfectly straight, and curve only in depth. A photograph taken from that point would be identical to a photograph taken in the real-world scene depicted in the diorama, i.e., the diorama and the scene it depicts share the same radial projection from the egocentric point (Lehar, 2003a,b). Fig. 6.5B shows an oblique view that makes the curvature more apparent. If you were to perceive this diorama the same way you normally perceive a real scene, you could ignore the perspective foreshortening and perceive the road to be straight and parallel and equidistant throughout its length, and the fence is perceived to be made of regular rectangles of equal size. If you perceive this diorama in that way, you would be seeing the diorama the same way that Eric Schwitzgebel views his own phenomenal perspective, and why he fails to notice any convergence at all, which is because our sense of size scale shrinks along with the road into the distance. What cannot be so easily ignored is the profound singularity where the parallel lines meet at "infinity," a point that is clearly less than an infinite distance away and the global warp of the whole space between the two vanishing points.

This "picture-in-the-head" or "Cartesian theatre" concept of visual representation has been criticized on the grounds that there would have to be a miniature observer to view this miniature internal scene, resulting in an infinite regress of observers within observers (Dennett, 1991, 1992;

O'Regan, 1992; Pessoa et al., 1998). In fact there is no need for an internal observer of the scene since the internal representation is simply a data structure like any other data in a computer, except that these data are expressed in spatial form (Earle, 1998; Singh and Hoffman, 1998; Lehar, 2003a). For if a picture in the head required a homunculus to view it, then the same argument would hold for any other form of information in the brain, which would also require a homunculus to read or interpret that information. In fact any information encoded in the brain needs only to be available to other internal processes rather than to a miniature copy of the whole brain. The fact that the brain does go to the trouble of constructing a full spatial analog of the external environment merely suggests that it has ways to make use of this spatial data. In any case the utility of being able to experience the visual world as a surrounding spatial structure is obvious to anyone who has had visual experience.

The failure of neuroscience to find any three-dimensional real-time moving colored images in the brain has prompted many to argue that it must be possible to have a three-dimensional extended experience without an explicit three-dimensional extended image-like representation in the brain. Max Velmans (1990) draws an analogy with a videotape recorder that records video images on a magnetic tape in a format that is not at all image-like, but more like a stream of abstract data that slices the image row-by-row and frame-by-frame. Information theory demonstrates that images can be compressed based on the redundancy they contain. An image of plain colored shapes can be compressed to an edge image to delimit the boundaries of each shape, with a single value to represent the color of each shape. Simple geometrical shapes can be reduced from a boundary to a formula for that shape, with a given location, orientation, and scale, so the formulas and their colors can be used to represent the whole image in compressed form. The consensus view in contemporary neuroscience is apparently that it is not necessary to look for images in the brain because a nonimage-like neural representation can correspond to an image-like experience. But this view is flawed based on information theory itself.

Although it is true that image information can be compressed to a compact nonspatial code, that code is useless without an image decompression algorithm that can read that compact code and reconstruct the original image when it is needed. The compression algorithm itself contains implicitly a lot of the information in the original image that was lost in the compression process, and that information can only be retrieved by the decompression algorithm that can restore the entire image with each pixel restored to its original color. In Max Velmans' videotape analogy, Velmans imagines the neural representation to be analogous to the abstract nonspatial information on the videotape, while the video image that it represents corresponds to our experience of the scene. But our experience, as an experience, is explicitly spatial, unlike the abstracted representation on the tape. Why would our experience not appear in the form that it is represented on the tape? What is it that performs the information-theoretic computation required to transform that abstract data back into the spatial image that we experience? The fact that our experience is image-like strongly implicates an explicit image-like representation in the brain. To deny the image-like nature of our visual experience is to deny its most prominent and significant properties. I propose that the spatial extendedness of visual experience, the fact that the color of colored surfaces is observed to pervade the entire colored surface, suggests that our visual experience is of an explicitly spatial reconstructed representation, not one that is compressed or abstracted to a nonspatial code. There is no question that some kind of simplification and compression is employed in the visual representation. But the rich edifice of visual consciousness *is* that simplified representation, it is immeasurably simplified relative to the real world that it represents, which we cannot see. But it is an explicitly spatial simplification that is experienced as a vivid spatial structure. If the idea of explicit spatial structures represented in the brain is inconsistent with contemporary concepts of neural computation, then it is our *theories of neural computation that are in urgent need of revision* because the evidence for the spatial nature of our visual representation is *primary* evidence, and thus more certain than anything modern neuroscience has discovered about the nature of visual consciousness.

Daniel Dennett (1991) argues that our experience is not at all as detailed and explicit as we experience it to be, that our experience is actually illusory. We *seem* to experience a lot more than we *actually* experience. But this is of course a contradiction in terms. Our experience is exactly as we experience it to be, and no different. While there is undoubtedly a considerable degree of compression and simplification in our perception of the world, our experience, as we experience it, *is* that compressed representation. It is not the original world that was the source of the light that entered our eye. And that compressed or abbreviated representation is expressed in the form of an explicit volumetric image that appears vividly realistic to us but is actually a highly simplified rendition of the world it depicts.

Information can exist in many different forms, from numbers printed on a page, to holes in punched cards, to magnetic domains on tape or disk. But in every case there must be a carrier, or medium, to carry the information. It is the modulations of that carrier, which record the information. And the same is true of perceptual or experiential information, such as the colored spatial world of our visual experience. Information theory suggests that the qualia of our experience, for example, the raw subjective experience of different colors, are the *carriers* of the information of our experience because it is the *modulation* of those carriers, such as the variation of color across space and time, which define the content of our visual experience. Information theory suggests therefore that the color in our experience is not the color of the world it represents, but a direct manifestation of the physical state of our brain that is used to represent color in the world. Locke's "primary qualities" of perception correspond to the information content of experience, whereas the "secondary qualities" are a direct manifestation of the mechanism that is modulated to express that information content.

6. CONCLUSION

The debate over the epistemology of visual experience has raged unresolved over many centuries, it is not likely to be resolved by this book. But this debate can be compared to a number of earlier debates that similarly challenged the materialistic view of the universe. Before Newton it was commonly thought that the heavens were fundamentally different than the earth, they were composed of different substance, and followed different laws. Since then we have discovered that the whole universe is made of the same kind of substance and follows the same laws. Before Darwin it was thought that human existence could not be explained without a supernatural intervention. The theory of natural selection showed how complexity can emerge from simplicity over a long period of time, and thus no invisible divine intervention was required to account for life. The theory of *animism*, popular in the last century, proposed that living organisms are more than just mere biochemistry, but that living things contained an *élan vitale*, a "vital essence" above and beyond biochemistry, and this vital essence, undetectable in principle, ceased to exist on the death of an organism without any corresponding change in its essential biochemistry. This too was another unfalsifiable hypothesis, whose prediction, that the *élan vitale* cannot be detected, is identical to the *null* prediction that the *élan vitale* does not exist.

The theory of direct perception is fundamentally flawed on epistemological grounds. It is impossible to even demonstrate the operational principle of direct perception in an artificial vision system, while the principle of representationalism is easily demonstrated with a video camera connected to a computer. Significantly, most proponents of direct perception believe that there is something magical in biological vision that cannot be replicated in an artificial vision system. There is no sense in which a photocell is "seeing" the light that it responds to electrically, they argue, it takes a living sentient creature to "see" anything at all. But this is just the latest case of mysticism masquerading as a scientific hypothesis, by people who cannot imagine how a mere mechanism could ever actually see. But for those of us who believe that we *are* biological automata, i.e., that there is no magic or mysticism in our existence or our consciousness, the fact that we can see already demonstrates that a biological automaton, made up of the ordinary substance of matter and energy, can see the world *as if* its experience were projecting out from its eyes into the world. It does not help in the least to attempt to "explain" this deep mystery by simply denying its existence and pretending that we can see directly, despite the evidence of our eyeballs, retina, and optic nerve to the brain, the mechanism of indirect sensory communication.

In the end this is a paradigm debate over whether vision is truly magical and beyond scientific explanation, or whether biological vision will eventually succumb to the ordinary scientific explanation of a physical process taking place in the physical mechanism of the brain. If science is to triumph over mysticism, the choice must be made based on the facts of the case, *regardless of the perceived incredibility* of the solution toward which all the facts point. Just that a theory *seems* incredible is not a valid argument to reject it. Indeed many of the greatest discoveries of science seemed initially to be so incredible that it took decades or even centuries before they were generally accepted. But accepted they were, eventually. And the reason why they were accepted was not because they had become any less incredible. Scientific fact is accepted on the basis of the evidence, regardless of the incredible truth to which that evidence points. Facts such as the immensity of the universe, and its cataclysmic genesis from a singularity in space and time, as well as the smallness of the atom, or the bizarre properties of quantum phenomena, are just as incredible today as they were when they were first proposed and yet all of these incredible theories have taken their place in the realm of accepted scientific knowledge not because they have become any less incredible since they were first proposed but because the *evidence for them has been irrefutable.* In science, irrefutable evidence triumphs over incredibility, and this is exactly what gives science the power to discover unexpected or incredible truth.

I am confident that the theory of direct perception, and its cognates in projection theory, and eliminative hypothesis will eventually be rejected as were their unfalsifiable precedents, and visual science will succumb, as all else has before it, to rational explanation in physical terms in a manner that will offer direct guidance as to how to devise an artificial vision system with the power of "external" perception (by way of an internal representation) that natural vision systems have enjoyed for millions of years.

REFERENCES

Broad, C.D., 1925. The Mind and Its Place in Nature. Routledge & Kegan Paul, London.

Dennett, D.C., 1991. Consciousness Explained. Little Brown & Co, Boston.

Dennett, D.C., 1992. 'Filling in' versus finding out: a ubiquitous confusion in cognitive science. In: Pick Jr., H.L., van den Broek, P., Knill, D.C. (Eds.), Cognition: Conceptual and Methodological Issues. American Psychological Association, Washington DC.

Drake, D., 1920. The approach to critical realism. In: Drake, D., Lovejoy, A.O., Pratt, J.B., Rogers, A.K., Santayana, G., Sellars, R.W., Strong, C.A. (Eds.), Essays in Critical Realism: A Co-operative Study of the Problem of Knowledge. Gordian Press, pp. 3–32.

Earle, D.C., 1998. On the roles of consciousness and representations in visual science. Behavioral & Brain Sciences 21 (6), 757–758. commentary on Pessoa et al. (1998).

Gibson, J.J., 1972. A theory of direct visual perception. In: Royce, J.R., Rozeboom, W.W. (Eds.), The Psychology of Knowing. Gordon & Breach.

Koffka, K., 1935. Principles of Gestalt Psychology. Harcourt Brace & Co, New York.

Köhler, W., Held, R., 1947. The cortical correlate of pattern vision. Science 110, 414–419.

Köhler, W., 1971. A task for philosophers. In: Henle, M. (Ed.), The Selected Papers of Wolfgang Koehler. Liveright, New York, pp. 83–107.

Lehar, S., 2003a. The World in Your Head: A Gestalt View of the Mechanism of Conscious Experience. Erlbaum, Mahwah NJ. Additional information at: http://cns-alumni. bu.edu/~slehar/webstuff/book/WIYH.html.

Lehar, S., 2003b. Gestalt isomorphism and the primacy of the subjective conscious experience: a gestalt bubble model. Behav. Brain Sci. 26 (4), 375–444. Also available at: http://cns-alumni.bu.edu/~slehar/webstuff/bubw3/bubw3.html.

Lehar, S., 1999. Hallway experiment. In: An Informal Experiment Conducted at the Schepens Eye Research Institute Documented on-line at: http://cns-alumni. bu.edu/~slehar/hallway/hallway.html (The outcome is so "obvious" that no formal experiment was really necessary, the reader can confirm the result for themself in any convenient hallway).

O'Regan, K.J., 1992. Solving the 'Real' mysteries of visual perception: the world as an outside memory. Can. J. Psychol. 46, 461–488.

Pastore, N., 1971. Selective History of Theories of Visual Perception. Oxford University Press, New York.

Pessoa, L., Thompson, E., Noë, A., 1998. Finding out about filling-in: a guide to perceptual completion for visual science and the philosophy of perception. Behav. Brain Sci. 21, 723–802.

Russell, B., 1921. The Analysis of Mind. George Allen & Unwin Ltd., New York. MacMilan, London.

Russell, B., 1927. Philosophy. W. W. Norton, New York.

Schwitzgebel, E., 2006. Do things look flat? Philos. Phenomenol. Res. 72 (3), 589–599.

Sellars, R. W., 1916. Critical Realism: A study of the Nature and Conditions of Knowledge. Russell & Russell, New York.

Singh, M., Hoffman, D.D., 1998. Active vision and the basketball problem Behavioral & Brain Sciences 21 (6), 772–773, commentary on Pessoa *et al.* (1998).

Smythies, J.R., 1989. The mind-brain problem. In: Smythies, J.R., Beloff, J. (Eds.), The Case for Dualism. University of Virginia Press, Charlottesville.

Smythies, J.R., 1994. The Walls of Plato's Cave: The Science and Philosophy of Brain, Consciousness, and Perception. Avebury, Aldershot UK.

Velmans, M., 1990. Consciousness, brain and the physical world. Philos. Psychol. 3 (1), 77–99.

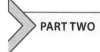

PART TWO

Papers Defending Direct Realism

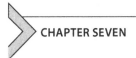

CHAPTER SEVEN

The Virtues of Direct Realism

Michael Huemer

Department of Philosophy, University of Colorado, Boulder, CO, United States

1. DIRECT AND INDIRECT REALISM

How do I know that my left foot exists? Because I can see it right now. Yes, but in what way does my seeing it give me justification for believing that the foot exists? There are two broad answers to this in the philosophical literature:

Direct Realism: Perception provides noninferential justification for external-world propositions.

Indirect Realism: Perception provides only inferential justification for external-world propositions.

In what follows, I shall explain why Direct Realism is a better theory than Indirect Realism.

But first, some clarification. What are external-world propositions? For present purposes, let us stipulate that external-world propositions are contingent propositions about the world independent of the mind. That is, they include things such as "There is a foot here" and "The sky is blue," but *not* such things as "Seven is more than five" (which is a necessary truth) or "I have a sensory appearance of a foot" (which is mind-dependent).

When I speak of the justification for external-world propositions provided by perception, I mean the justification provided in normal, favorable cases of perception. I do not assume that perception *always* provides justification; perhaps there are special cases in which it does not. For example, if a person mistakenly thinks that he is hallucinating, then perhaps his perception fails to justify external-world claims for him. I do assume, however, that perception sometimes provides justification for external-world beliefs; that is, I assume skepticism is false. Direct Realists hold that *at least some* external-world propositions are non-inferentially justified. Indirect Realists hold that some external-world propositions are inferentially justified, and *none* are noninferentially justified.

What is meant by "inferential justification"? The paradigm of inferential justification is the kind of justification one has for a belief when one

Direct versus Indirect Realism
ISBN 978-0-12-812141-2
https://doi.org/10.1016/B978-0-12-812141-2.00007-6

explicitly, consciously reasons to that belief, starting from other beliefs that are justified. But to be fair to Indirect Realists, we should not saddle them with the incredible view that all justified external-world beliefs are justified by conscious reasoning from other beliefs. Everyone (except the skeptics) knows that is false. We should therefore allow the Indirect Realist to introduce weaker notions of inferential justification. For instance, a belief may qualify as inferentially justified if it is arrived at through unconscious or implicit inference. In addition, to be generous to Indirect Realists, let us allow that a belief may count as inferentially justified, provided that its justification depends on the subject's *having justification for* some other proposition.

Here is an example. I am at the airport, heading for an international flight. A security guard asks me my country of residence. "I live in the United States," I answer. The skeptical guard asks, "And what' your justification for believing that?" An odd question, to be sure, but what is the answer?

I would not say that I have inferred that I live in the United States from some premises—certainly not at the time I was just asked, and possibly not ever.[1] Even if I did originally acquire the belief by an inference, which has little to do with my present justification since I know that I live in the United States regardless of whether my original reason for adopting this belief (back when I was a very young child) was a good one. But the belief is not independent of the rest of my belief system: I could not justifiedly believe that I live in the United States unless I had some other beliefs. As a matter of fact, I have a host of background knowledge about my life and about the United States that would make it irrational for me to doubt that I live in the United States.

Let us agree to count this sort of belief as inferentially justified. That is, a belief will count as inferentially justified, for our purposes, provided that its justification depends on the subject's having justification for some other beliefs.

The Indirect Realist claims that this is true of all external-world beliefs, including perceptual beliefs: even when I see my foot right in front of me, says the Indirect Realist, my justification for believing that the foot exists depends on my having justification for some other beliefs. What other beliefs? Traditionally, Indirect Realists think that our justification for claims about the external world always depends on our justification for one or more propositions about mind-dependent phenomena—sensations, "sense data,"

---

[1] This example is from Leite (2008, pp. 434–435).

states of being appeared to, etc. So my justification for thinking my foot exists depends on my justification for thinking that a footlike sense datum exists (or that I have a sensory experience representing a foot, or that there appears to me to be a foot, or something similar). In addition, we allegedly need justification for taking these mind-dependent phenomena to be correlated in certain ways with phenomena in the physical world.

Direct Realists need neither deny that such mind-dependent phenomena exist nor deny that we can have justified beliefs about them. What Direct Realists deny is that our justification for claims about the external world *depends on* justification for claims about something mind-dependent. They think that the starting points of our knowledge and reasoning may include certain facts about the world outside our minds.

My account of Direct and Indirect Realism here is exclusively epistemological: both views concern how we acquire knowledge or justification. There are other senses of "Direct Realism" and "Indirect Realism" (for instance, one on which the issue concerns the objects of "direct awareness" or "direct perception"). These other notions of Direct and Indirect Realism are perfectly reasonable and interesting things to discuss, but they are not my focus here.[2]

2. A VERSION OF DIRECT REALISM

2.1 Phenomenal Conservatism

I have elsewhere defended a general theory about the justification for beliefs known as "Phenomenal Conservatism."[3] The theory holds that a person has justification for believing that P, provided that (1) it seems to them that P, and (2) they have no reason for doubting this appearance. In other words, there is a rational presumption that things are the way they appear; if a skeptic wants us to doubt the appearances, the skeptic has a burden of providing grounds for doubt. This theory applies to all kinds of beliefs, whether acquired by perception, memory, introspection, or intuition—all are rendered justified by appearances (in the absence of grounds for doubt); in fact, there is nothing else that could serve as an ultimate source of justification for anything. The theory applies even to inferential beliefs: an argument can provide justification for believing its conclusion only if the premises seem

---

[2] For discussion of issues about direct awareness, see my 2001, Ch. 4.
[3] Huemer (2001, Ch. 5, 2006, 2007). For critical discussion of the theory, see the selections in Tucker (2013).

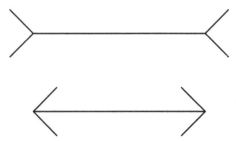

Figure 7.1 The Müller-Lyer illusion.

to support the conclusion and the premises seem correct (or seem to be supported by further premises that seem correct, etc.).

Since I have given general arguments for Phenomenal Conservatism elsewhere, I will not repeat them here. Instead, I will simply turn to what a phenomenal conservative should say about perception.

2.2 The Justification of Perceptual Beliefs

During normal perception, one has a kind of experience called a "perceptual experience." Perceptual experiences inherently represent the world around one as being a certain way; that is, they have representational content. At least some of this content is independent of the perceiver's beliefs. For example, in the famous Müller-Lyer illusion (Fig. 7.1), the top line looks longer than the bottom line, regardless of what one believes. Even for subjects who know for certain that the lines are the same length, the top line still looks longer. We might say that one has a visual experience representing the top line as longer, which is not dependent on background beliefs or knowledge and may in fact conflict with one's background knowledge. This visual experience, such as all perceptual experiences, is an appearance state: that is, a mental state whereby it seems to one that the world is a certain way.

According to Phenomenal Conservatism, one is justified in believing the contents of one's perceptual experiences—believing that the world is the way it seems to be—by default, provided that one has no particular grounds for doubt. The contents of our perceptual experiences are external-world propositions, not propositions about our minds, or anything dependent on the mind. For example, when I see my foot, my visual experience represents that there is a foot there; it does not represent that there is a mental state. In other words, what immediately seems to me to be the case, by virtue of my having this experience, is *that there is a foot*; what seems to me to be the case is not that there is a footlike sense datum, or a collection of sensations, or an appearance of a foot. So what I am justified in believing, according

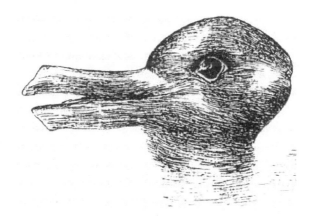

Figure 7.2 The duck rabbit.

to Phenomenal Conservatism, is an external-world proposition, in this case that there is a foot.

What sort of justification is this: inferential or noninferential? According to Phenomenal Conservatism, appearances are an intrinsic, ultimate source of justification. In the absence of defeaters, the appearance that P suffices for P to be justified, and no further beliefs, awareness, or other mental states are required. A subject does not, for example, require the additional belief that appearances are generally true or independent evidence for the reliability of appearances; it simply is rational to start from the way things seem, by default. Sensory appearances, then, provide noninferential justification for external-world propositions.

2.3 The Cognitive Mediation of Perceptual Content

Some aspects of our perceptual experiences depend on background knowledge and experience. Thus, consider the ambiguous image in Fig. 7.2, which can be viewed alternately as a duck or a rabbit.[4] A subject who had previous awareness only of ducks could only see Fig. 7.2 as a duck image; one who had awareness only of rabbits could only see it as a rabbit image. Those with previous awareness of both can switch between the two ways of seeing the image. The switch in ways of seeing the image is not a switch in any *beliefs* one has; it is genuinely a switch in ways of perceiving the image. This illustrates that how we perceive what is in front of us—and thus, what seems

---

[4] The image is taken from Jastrow (1899, p. 312), who credits the magazine *Fliegende Blätter*.

to us to be the case when we have perceptual experiences—can depend in certain respects on our past experience and knowledge.

One might consider this phenomenon to challenge Direct Realism in some sense since it shows that our perceptual awareness is mediated by background knowledge. Of course, the "in some sense" qualifier here is crucial. The only sense of "Direct Realism" at issue in this chapter is the epistemological sense defined in Section 1: Direct Realism as the thesis that perception provides noninferential justification for some external-world propositions. Keeping that sense in mind, does the cognitive mediation of perceptual content pose a problem for Direct Realism?

The answer is no, for two reasons. First, recall that Direct Realism does not claim that all external-world propositions can be noninferentially justified; it only claims that there are some external-world propositions that receive noninferential justification during normal perceptual experiences. Indirect Realists must argue that there are no such propositions. A thesis that applies only to some of the content of perceptual experiences could not refute Direct Realism. And this is the case for the cognitive mediation thesis: only certain aspects of perceptual experience depend on background knowledge. Only those with knowledge or experience of ducks can see the duck aspect of the image in Fig. 7.2. Only those with knowledge or experience pertaining to rabbits can see the rabbit aspect. But everyone can see a certain very specific shape on the page, whether or not they see that shape as representing some kind of animal or other object. This is to say that part of the content of one's perceptual experience depends on background knowledge or experience, and part of it does not. Furthermore, it could not possibly be that all perceptual content depends on background knowledge or experience because if that were so, then there would have been no way to acquire background knowledge or experience to begin with. I assume that we neither have a priori knowledge of the external world nor do we have an infinite series of experiences going back forever; therefore, there must be a time when human beings *start* to perceive phenomena in the external world (properties, states of affairs, types of objects, etc.). This could never happen if all perception depended on background knowledge of the external world.

Here is the second reason why cognitive mediation is not a problem for Direct Realism: Direct and Indirect Realism are theses about epistemic justification, that is, about what makes beliefs rational or reasonable, or why it makes sense to hold certain beliefs. To defend Indirect Realism, what one has to argue is not that the contents of perceptual experiences causally depend on past experience, knowledge, or concepts. What one has to argue is that the *justification* for perceptual *beliefs* always depends on the justification for some other propositions. And that thesis is not supported by the phenomenon of cognitive mediation of perceptual content. In short, the putative challenge to Direct Realism is aimed at a mistaken target.

3. THE BASING PROBLEM

3.1 The Indirect Realist's Case for an External World

The preceding discussion should give some idea of why I find epistemological Direct Realism plausible; the theory fits with my general account of justified belief. But here I want to discuss the advantages of Direct Realism in accounting specifically for perceptual knowledge, whatever one thinks about the rest of human knowledge.

The most obvious problem for Indirect Realism as an epistemological theory is the basing problem. The problem is that Indirect Realist accounts of the justification for external-world propositions threaten to put that justification beyond the reach of ordinary, unsophisticated subjects—including not just animals and children, but perhaps all but a handful of the human beings who have ever lived. On Indirect Realist accounts, we may have some source of justification *available* for external-world propositions, but our actual beliefs will neither be justified nor will they qualify as knowledge because our beliefs are not in fact based on the good reasons that we have available.

According to most Indirect Realists, the justification for external-world propositions derives from an inference to the best explanation: the hypothesis of a real world—filled with physical objects that we can perceive and that continue to exist when are not looking at them—provides the best explanation for why we have the sensory experiences (these being purely internal mental states) that we in fact have.

Why is this the best explanation? Why not hypothesize instead that we are brains in vats, or that a powerful demon is planting false images in our minds? One argument is that these alternative explanations are inferior because they are more complex because they have to rely on ad hoc posits to explain why the objects we seem to perceive obey the principles that real physical objects would have to obey.[5] For example, according to Jonathan Vogel, it is a priori impossible for real, solid objects to occupy the same place at the same time. But it is not in principle impossible for a *simulation* to

[5] Vogel (2014).

represent objects as occupying the same place at the same time. Therefore, to explain why we do not observe physical objects coinciding in space, the brain-in-a-vat theory would have to introduce extra, contingent stipulations of a sort that the real-world theory does not require. This makes the brain-in-a-vat theory inferior to the real-world theory.

Another argument is that the alternative hypotheses are inferior because they make much less specific predictions than the real-world hypothesis.[6] For example, the real-world theory predicts that we should have generally coherent experiences, experiences that can be seen as accurately representing stable physical objects obeying consistent laws of nature. The brain-in-a-vat theory, by contrast, is compatible with any possible sequence of experiences, whether coherent or not. There is no particular reason why the scientists stimulating a brain in a vat need to give the brain coherent experiences. Since the overwhelming majority of possible sequences of experiences are incoherent (e.g., random mixtures of colors, sounds, and so on), the probability of our having coherent experiences given the brain-in-a-vat theory is close to zero. Therefore, our actual coherent experiences render it highly probable that we are perceiving the real world.

3.2 The Basing Problem

Suppose that some such argument is correct. Still, it seems clear that these arguments have nothing to do with why ordinary people actually believe what they do about the external world. When a normal person sees a marmot, he does not go through anything like the reasoning alluded to above, not even unconsciously or implicitly. He does not think to himself, "Well, I'm having a marmot-representing sensory experience right now. I wonder what could be causing it. Let me list the alternative explanations and the theoretical virtues and vices of each... Okay, it looks like the real-world theory wins out. So there is most likely an actual marmot in front of me." It is not just that he does not rehearse that reasoning at the time he sees the marmot; most people have *never* gone through any reasoning at all like that. Most have never entertained alternative explanations for their sensory experiences—and even among those who have (such as students in introductory philosophy classes), most have no idea of how to argue against the alternatives.

---

[6] Huemer (2016). Although I endorse this as an argument against skeptical scenarios, I do not claim either that it has anything to do with why most people hold the beliefs that they do or therefore that it does explain our actual knowledge.

Why does this matter? It matters because of a principle known as *the Basing Requirement* for knowledge or justified belief. The principle is that a person counts as knowing or justifiedly believing P only if he believes P for the right reasons (that is, for some rational reasons). In other words, it is not enough that I have some justification for P available to me; I must also in fact base my belief that P on the thing that provides that justification.

Here is an example to illustrate the Basing Requirement. Ted is an evangelical Christian. For many years, Ted has refused to accept the theory of evolution because he does not want to believe that his ancestors were monkeys. This is despite the fact that, let us suppose, Ted has plenty of compelling evidence of the theory's truth: he knows about the fossil record, about the morphological similarities among organisms of different species, the evidence of vestigial physiological structures in certain organisms, and so on. Ted does not care about any of that evidence. One day, however, Ted visits a psychic who, after looking into a crystal ball, declares that the theory of evolution is true. Ted thereupon finally accepts the theory of evolution, solely because of the psychic's announcement (he still does not care about the scientific evidence). Question: does Ted have a justified belief in the theory of evolution?

Intuitively, what we should say is that although Ted *has justification available* for the theory (he knows the scientific evidence that supports it), his actual belief is unjustified since it is not based on any of that evidence. It is based on the psychic's testimony, which is not an adequate source of evidence. In short, Ted believes the right thing for the wrong reason. He also thereby falls short of *knowing* that the theory of evolution is true.

If Indirect Realism is true, something similar is true of virtually all of us, with respect to our beliefs about the external world: we have good reasons available to us but since we do not believe on the basis of those reasons, our actual beliefs would be unjustified, and we would not count as actually *knowing* anything about the external world. This, I take it, is an extremely undesirable consequence for an epistemological theory.

3.3 The Broad Notion of Inferential Justification

To return to a point from Section 1 above, we should not interpret inferential justification too narrowly. When I say that I live in the United States, it is also true that I never actually reasoned to that conclusion. I never entertained alternative theories about where I might be living, never came up with an argument that I am not really living on the Sun, etc. Nevertheless, we do not want to say that the belief that I live in the United States is unjustified (nor is it noninferentially justified). As we have said, the belief counts as inferentially justified because it depends for its justification on background knowledge that I have about the United States and about my general biography. Why cannot the Indirect Realist say that our perceptual beliefs work similarly: they are justified even though we never went through the reasoning that supports them? How do ordinary people's perceptual beliefs about the external world differ from my belief that I live in the United States?

I think there are two important differences. First, the background information that would be said to support the belief that I live in the United States is information that I definitely believe or at one time believed. For example, I believe that I live in Denver, that Denver is the capitol of Colorado, and that Colorado is a US state. The last time I flew on an airplane, it was to return to Denver; at the time, I saw a screen listing where the flight to Denver was boarding, and I went to that gate. Before takeoff, the flight crew announced over the public address system (PA) that this was such-and-such flight number, to Denver. These are all things that I was most definitely aware of, and they are all part of the evidence that I live in the United States.

By contrast, the arguments that are said to justify my belief in the external world include premises or ways of reasoning that ordinary people do not presently endorse and have never endorsed, even dispositionally. For instance, to justify the belief that my left foot exists, philosophers such as Vogel would say, among other things:
1. The brain-in-a-vat theory requires ad hoc postulates to explain why we do not experience external objects as colocated.
2. This renders the brain-in-a-vat theory more complex than the real-world theory.
3. Other things being equal, more complex theories are less probable than simpler theories.

This is all, allegedly, essential to the justification for my belief about the foot since an inference to the best explanation must rule out alternative explanations. But it is extremely farfetched to ascribe all those beliefs to an ordinary person. (I, of course, am a special case since I am familiar with the philosophical literature. Maybe *I* believe those things, but typical nonphilosophers do not.) Many people, if asked whether all those things are true, would shrug their shoulders. Many would have trouble even understanding the claims being made; among those who understood the claims, many would have trouble deciding whether they were true. It is still more absurd to suggest, say, that a cat or a five-year-old child holds those beliefs. But cats and children know things about the world around them.

Here is the second difference between perceptual beliefs and my belief that I live in the United States: the other beliefs and experiences that could be said to justify my belief that I live in the United States can, taken collectively, be plausibly ascribed *some causal role* in supporting that belief.

> I say "taken collectively" because it may seem that no one belief or experience is causally relevant by itself. For example, today I found a bill in my mailbox. It was addressed to me, and the address included the phrase, "Denver, CO." This is evidence that I live in Denver, Colorado—but of course, by itself this experience had no detectable impact on my opinions about where I live. If the address had named a city in Slovenia, I would not have changed my mind about my residence; I would merely have concluded that the post office had made a hilarious error. I have, however, had a great many experiences of this sort, experiences that fit together with the idea that I live in the United States and what is important is that as a whole, this body of experience is causally relevant to my belief that I live in the United States: if I had never had any experiences like that—if the address on my mail never named a US city, if I never heard people around me talking about the United States as their country, and so on—then I would not now be so confident that I live in the United States In this admittedly weak sense, my belief that I live in the United States is **based on** those experiences.

By contrast, it is not plausible at all to say that my belief that my left foot exists is in fact based—even in a weak sense—on the sort of reasoning Indirect Realists appeal to. In no sense is it true that I believe in external objects *because of* that reasoning. If I did not accept the sort of premises mentioned above, I would nonetheless confidently accept the existence of the external objects I perceive around me. Even if I thought every Indirect Realist argument for the existence of external objects failed, I would still believe, with near-total confidence that the physical objects I seem to perceive exist. I think most people are like me in this respect.

3.4 The Direct Realist Alternative

So the Indirect Realist has trouble explaining how ordinary people qualify as knowing or justifiedly believing propositions about the external world. The Direct Realist, by contrast, has no problem granting external-world knowledge to typical adults, as well as children and animals. On my account, the justification for external-world propositions derives directly from appearances, with no auxiliary premises needed. To have a justified belief that my left foot exists, all I have to do is have an experience in which the foot seems to me to exist, with no reasons for doubting its existence, and that experience must cause me to think the foot exists. The Basing Requirement poses no problem since appearances provide eminently plausible explanations for what actually causes our beliefs. Indeed, even a baby marmot can acquire justified external-world beliefs, on a Direct Realist account.

4. THE SYMMETRY ARGUMENT

4.1 The Asymmetry in Indirect Realism

In this section, I want to point out a feature of Indirect Realism that makes it theoretically fishy, beyond the basing problem mentioned in the last section. The Indirect Realist must posit an asymmetry between different classes of appearances, an asymmetry that lacks clear motivation. That is, the view that the Indirect Realist takes of sensory appearances is not one that he could take about appearances in general, but there is no obvious reason why sensory appearances should be epistemologically different from nonsensory appearances. The most theoretically natural approach would treat sensory and nonsensory appearances alike, as Direct Realists do.

The Indirect Realist denies that a perceptual experience as of P, by itself, gives one any justification at all, even in the absence of defeaters, for believing that P. Why? What more do Indirect Realists think that one needs? Generally speaking, they think that one needs some evidence, or reasons for believing, that sensory experiences are reliable indicators of facts in the external world—that marmot experiences tend to be caused by marmots, foot experiences by feet, and so on. To be sure, they think we in fact have such evidence, so we are in fact justified in our external-world beliefs, but this justification is inferential, not immediate.

This view about perception could not be applied consistently across modes of awareness or cognitive faculties. The view requires us to start out distrusting our senses and then establish knowledge of their reliability using other cognitive faculties or belief-forming methods. To justify external-world propositions, we allegedly must construct an inference to the best explanation, which requires the use of (1) introspection, to identify the data that needs to be explained; (2) intellectual intuition, to identify the criteria for best explanations; (3) reasoning; and (4) memory, to retain knowledge during the reasoning process of what was established earlier in the reasoning. These four other types of awareness or belief formation cannot themselves be treated in the same manner as perception, or else we shall be embarked on an infinite regress. If, that is, we are to also start out distrusting each of these other cognitive faculties, and if we must verify *their* reliability before we may rely on them, then we shall have nowhere to start.

The Indirect Realist, then, owes us some account of the asymmetry: why is the default attitude toward perception different from the default attitude toward beliefs formed by other means? Thomas Reid, writing 250 years ago, put the problem thus:

The skeptic asks me, why do you believe the existence of the external object which you perceive? This belief, sir, is none of my manufacture; it came from the mint of nature; it bears her image and superscription; and, if it is not right, the fault is not mine: I even took it on trust, and without suspicion. Reason, says the skeptic, is the only judge of truth, and you ought to throw off every opinion and every belief that is not grounded on reason. Why, sir, should I believe the faculty of reason more than that of perception?—they came both out of the same shop and were made by the same artist; and if he puts one piece of false ware into my hands, what should hinder him from putting another?[7]

4.2 Accounting for Asymmetry: Vulnerability to Error

One account of the asymmetry comes from Descartes: perceptual beliefs are capable of being mistaken, or it is possible to have grounds for doubting them, whereas beliefs about our present, conscious mental states, and beliefs in simple necessary truths cannot be mistaken, and it is not possible to have grounds for doubting them.[8] For example, the possibility that you may be dreaming right now casts doubt on your perceptual beliefs. But it does not cast doubt on your beliefs about your current mental states or about simple necessary truths since these beliefs would still be true even if you were dreaming. Therefore, Descartes thought, perceptual beliefs require support of a kind that introspective beliefs and beliefs about simple necessary truths do not.

There are two problems with this reasoning. The first is that the premise is false: introspective beliefs and beliefs about simple necessary truths are not immune to error. It is possible, for example, to introspectively believe that one is feeling indignation and a desire for justice, when one is merely feeling envy. It is possible to introspectively believe that one is in pain, when in fact one has only a discomfort that is very close to the threshold for counting as a pain.[9] It is possible to mistakenly intuit that the Comprehension Axiom of naïve set theory is true, viz., that for any

---

[7] Reid ([1764] 1997, section 6.20, pp. 168–169).

[8] Descartes ([1641] 1984), Meditations 1–2.

[9] Williamson (2002, pp. 96–98) uses cases of this sort to show that we do not necessarily know the present, conscious mental states we are in.

predicate there is a set containing all and only the things satisfying that predicate. Indeed, most people who think about set theory have precisely that intuition, which presents itself as the intuition of a simple, necessary truth. In fact, the Comprehension Axiom is a necessary falsehood. And of course, it is perfectly possible to have grounds for doubting these sorts of things, as when Bertrand Russell presented his infamous paradox, refuting the Comprehension Axiom.

The second problem with the "vulnerability to error/grounds for doubt" account is that the conclusion is simply a nonsequitur. From the premise that some class of beliefs are capable of being mistaken, it simply does not follow that those beliefs are not foundational, i.e., noninferentially justified. "Noninferential" does not mean "infallible"; it means "not dependent on other justified propositions." It appears that Descartes simply confused these two quite different attributes that a belief might have. In the case of mathematical systems, which Descartes took as a sort of model for human knowledge in general, the two attributes go together: the axioms from which a mathematical system starts are typically both noninferentially justified and infallible, or something close to it. But there is no reason why these two attributes must always coincide—no reason why a system of beliefs cannot contain fallible starting points.

A similar point applies to the notion of grounds for doubt. To be noninferentially justified, a belief must have a justification not derived from the justification for any other propositions; it does not follow from this that other justified propositions could not in the future undermine its justification. Where a belief's justification came from and what might undermine it are two different questions.

4.3 Kinds of Error

Another idea for the Indirect Realist is that, even if all kinds of belief are subject to error in one way or another, perceptual beliefs are vulnerable to certain kinds of error to which introspective and intuitive beliefs are not, and as a result, perceptual beliefs can never be *as* certain as the most secure introspective and intuitive beliefs.

The concern about levels of certainty here is simply another iteration of the confusion between a belief's *degree* of justification and the belief's *source* of justification. There is no reason why noninferential sources would have to produce a higher degree of justification than inferential sources.

The claim about kinds of error is true: there are ways in which perception can go wrong that do not apply to other belief-forming methods. If, for example, one is a brain in a vat, then one's perceptual beliefs are massively in error, yet one's introspective and intuitive beliefs are most likely still perfectly reliable. But the conclusion that perceptual beliefs are not foundational is, again, a nonsequitur. It is probably true of every belief-forming method that there are ways it can go wrong that do not apply to other methods. Thus, the belief in the naïve Comprehension Axiom is mistaken—and however, we want to describe how that belief goes wrong, it seems that perceptual beliefs cannot go wrong in *that* way. But this does not show that intuitive beliefs cannot be noninferentially justified.

4.4 Acquaintance

Here is a third account of the crucial difference between perceptual beliefs and intuitive or introspective beliefs: in the case of intuitive or introspective beliefs, one may be *acquainted with* the facts that make them true, whereas this is not true of perceptual beliefs. Acquaintance, in this view, is a kind of irreducible, direct awareness. This is a factive mental state, that is, a mental state whose occurrence logically entails the existence of its object.

But why think that perceptual beliefs are not supported by acquaintance—why cannot perception constitute this sort of direct awareness of external objects? Richard Fumerton gives an argument appealing to the possibility of a fully convincing, vivid, and detailed hallucination:

1. In the case of a perfectly realistic hallucination as of P, one has the same sort of justification for believing P as one has when one perceives that P.
2. When one hallucinates that P, one's justification for believing P does not consist of one's acquaintance with the fact that P since one is not in fact so acquainted.
3. Therefore, when one perceives that P, one's justification for believing that P also does not consist of one's acquaintance with the fact that P[10].

Suppose one thinks (as Fumerton does) that all noninferential justification derives from direct acquaintance. Then it follows that perception does not provide noninferential justification.

My response: Fumerton's argument does not evince a real asymmetry between perception and other cognitive faculties because a parallel argument can be constructed for other forms of cognition. Take the case of a mistaken intellectual intuition, such as the intuition that the naïve Comprehension Axiom is true. The following argument strikes me as equally plausible as Fumerton's argument:

---

[10] Fumerton (1985, pp. 78ff).

1. In the case of a mistaken intuition that P, one has the same sort of justification for believing P as one has when one correctly intuits that P.
2. When one mistakenly intuits that P, one's justification for believing P does not consist of one's acquaintance with the fact that P.
3. Therefore, when one correctly intuits that P, one's justification for believing that P also does not consist of one's acquaintance with the fact that P.

A parallel argument can be constructed for mistaken introspective judgments and mistaken memories, showing that in none of these cases does one's justification for belief derive from acquaintance.

I think the proper conclusion to draw is not that none of these cognitive faculties provide noninferential justification or knowledge. The proper conclusion to draw is that noninferential justification and knowledge do not require acquaintance. Instead, they rest on appearances.

5. CONCLUSION

Direct Realists hold that when we normally perceive external objects, we thereby acquire justification for believing that these objects exist and are as they appear, and this justification does not essentially depend on our having justification for any other propositions. Indirect Realists, by contrast, hold that our justification for beliefs about the objects that we perceive essentially depends on our justification for certain other propositions—especially propositions describing our mental states and propositions attributing a reliable correlation between certain mental states and certain states of the physical world. The justification for believing in such correlations, in turn, is supposed to rest on an inference in which it is shown that the hypothesis of a real world corresponding to our sensory experiences provides the best explanation for the character of our experiences.

Direct Realism is a better epistemological theory than Indirect Realism, for two main reasons. The first is that Indirect Realists cannot plausibly explain how ordinary people, ignorant of sophisticated philosophical theories, possess justified beliefs and knowledge of the external world. This is because ordinary people do not, even in the broadest sense, base their beliefs about the external world on anything remotely like what philosophers say would justify those beliefs.

The second reason why Direct Realism is superior is that Indirect Realists have to posit an asymmetry between perception and other cognitive faculties: the rational default attitude, they say, is to be distrustful of perception until one acquires positive evidence that perception is reliable—but the Indirect Realists do not think the same is true of intellectual intuition, introspection, or memory (and if they did, they would be forced into skepticism). But there is no good reason for positing such an asymmetry. All cognitive faculties, not just perception, are fallible, and while perception is capable of going wrong in ways that do not apply to introspection or intuition, this fact is irrelevant to the issue of noninferential justification. The fact that perceptual beliefs are fallible and may be rationally revised does not preclude their being justified noninferentially. The Indirect Realists are correct to deny that perceptual beliefs are justified by acquaintance. However, this fails to establish an asymmetry between perception and other cognitive faculties because no beliefs are justified by acquaintance. The same sort of argument can be given for all cognitive faculties: there are cases of justified but mistaken beliefs of each type (perceptual, introspective, intuitive, mnemonic) that seem to be justified in the same way as paradigmatic correct beliefs. So this justification cannot derive from some condition that guarantees the belief's truth.

Direct Realism avoids the problems facing Indirect Realism. Direct Realists can explain the justification of perceptual beliefs by appealing to the principle of Phenomenal Conservatism, namely, that it is rational in general to begin with the presumption that things are the way they seem, unless and until one acquires specific reasons for thinking otherwise. Direct Realists can easily account for the ordinary person's knowledge of the external world since ordinary people base their external-world beliefs on appearances, just as (according to Phenomenal Conservatism) one should. Direct realists need posit no asymmetry among our cognitive faculties since the principle of Phenomenal Conservatism applies equally to all appearances: whether we are considering perceptual, introspective, mnemonic, or intuitive appearances, it makes sense to assume that things are the way they appear in the absence of specific grounds for doubt.

REFERENCES

Descartes, R., [1641] 1984. In: Cottingham, J., Stoothoff, R., Murdoch, D., Meditations on First Philosophy in the Philosophical Writings of Descartes, vol. 2. Cambridge University Press, Cambridge.

Fumerton, R., 1985. Metaphysical and Epistemological Problems of Perception. University of Nebraska Press, Lincoln, Nebr.

Huemer, M., 2001. Skepticism and the Veil of Perception. Rowman & Littlefield, Lanham, MD.

Huemer, M., 2006. Phenomenal conservatism and the internalist intuition. Am. Philos. Q. 43, 147–158.

Huemer, M., 2007. Compassionate phenomenal conservatism. Philos. Phenomenol. Res. 74, 30–55.

Huemer, M., 2016. Serious Theories and Skeptical Theories: Why You Are Probably Not a Brain in a Vat. 173. Philosophical Studies, pp. 1031–1052.

Jastrow, J., 1899. The mind's eye. Popular Sci. Mon. 54, 299–312.

Leite, A., 2008. Believing one's reasons are good. Synthese 161, 419–441.

Reid, T., [1764] 1997. In: Brookes, D.R. (Ed.), An Inquiry into the Human Mind on the Principles of Common Sense. Pennsylvania State University Press. University Park.

Tucker, C., 2013. Seemings and Justification: New Essays on Dogmatism and Phenomenal Conservatism. Oxford University Press, Oxford.

Vogel, J., 2014. The refutation of skepticism. In: Steup, M., Turri, J., Sosa, E. (Eds.), Contemporary Debates in Epistemology, second ed. Wiley-Blackwell, Malden, Mass, pp. 108–120.

Williamson, T., 2002. Knowledge and Its Limits. Oxford University Press, Oxford.

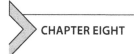

CHAPTER EIGHT

Direct Realism, Disjunctivism, and Screening Off

William Fish
Philosophy Department, Massey University, Palmerston North, New Zealand

In this paper, I begin by exploring the ways in which John Foster attempts to articulate the key distinction between direct and indirect perception. I argue that neither of these approaches succeeds in developing a philosophically substantive conception of the key notion of direct access. Against this background, I offer a new way of understanding the key notion of direct—and hence also indirect—access in terms of phenomenal mediation. In the second half of the paper I turn to exploring what constraints this understanding of the direct/indirect distinction places on theories that aspire to qualify as versions of direct realism. I argue that any theory that qualifies as providing direct access must be a form of disjunctivism and, more substantially, a form of negative disjunctivism that places significant restrictions on the philosophical theory we can offer of those cases that are not themselves perceptual in nature, yet are introspectively indiscriminable from perceptual experiences of a certain kind. Nothing in this paper will constitute an argument for negative disjunctivism, however—merely a conditional claim that, if one wants a theory of perception that provides for a philosophically substantive direct access to mind-independent reality, then one will need to be a negative disjunctivist.

1. PART I: THE DIRECT/INDIRECT DISTINCTION

As it is typically understood, the group of theories that we would classify as "direct realist" theories have two key components: *realism* about the nature of the physical world—that is, that it exists independently of human (or indeed any) minds—alongside the idea that, in perception, we have *direct access* to that world. Direct realism's counterpart—*indirect* realism—agrees on the realism but disagrees on the claim about our access to that world. The focus of the present paper will thus be on that of direct versus indirect access.

Direct versus Indirect Realism
ISBN 978-0-12-812141-2
https://doi.org/10.1016/B978-0-12-812141-2.00008-8

Before we begin, however, I want to briefly consider why, when developing a philosophical theory of perception, it was deemed necessary to say *anything* explicit about the nature of our access to the mind-independent world. To see why this became important, consider what Locke says about perception as an example of early modern thinking on the subject. On one interpretation of Locke's claim that it is "the actual receiving of ideas from without that gives us notice of the existence of other things" (Locke, 1961; Book 4, Ch.11, §2), the "ideas" that we receive are actually objects in themselves, distinct from the mind-independent objects that populate the realist's world. Yet if the redness that characterizes my perception of a cherry is a quality of an *idea*, rather than of the cherry itself, then this can make it look as though, although we naturally take ourselves to see a (mind-independent) cherry, what we *really*—strictly speaking—see is in fact merely an *idea* that resembles a cherry. Although it is not clear that Locke himself held this view, it nonetheless clearly displays the underlying concern that on some theories of perception, there will be a "veil of perception" (Bennett, 1971, p. 69) that will function as "an interface between our cognitive powers and the external world – or, to put the same point differently, ... that our cognitive powers cannot reach all the way to the objects themselves" (Putnam, 1994, p. 453). The underlying worry is thus that some theories of perception seem to posit something that functions as a veil or interface, which acts so as to screen off or block our cognitive powers from reaching all the way to the world. When we distinguish between direct and indirect modes of access to the mind-independent world, what we are thus trying to capture is the distinction between theories that incorporate such an interface and theories that allow our cognitive powers to "reach all the way to the objects themselves."

In *The Nature of Perception*, John Foster discusses two ways in which we might draw the distinction between what is involved in having "direct access" to mind-independent objects and what would be the case if our access to such objects were merely indirect. Foster's first characterization of the direct/indirect distinction turns on the idea of *perceptual mediation*: S's perception of one object—x—is *mediated* when the fact of S's perceiving x is constituted by S's perceiving of some other object, y, and certain additional facts. To explain this notion of perceptual mediation, Foster discusses the sense in which Pauline's perceiving an apple (x) is constituted by her perceiving the apple's front surface (y) together with the fact that the surface she sees is a portion of the apple's surface. Other examples could include one's perceiving the following vehicle (x) being constituted by one's perceiving the reflection in the mirror (y), plus the fact that y is a reflection of x; or that one's perceiving a temporally extended event (x) is constituted by one's perceiving the component of x that is taking place *now* (y) plus the fact that y is a temporal part of x.

With this definition in mind, consider what Foster calls Φ-terminal perceiving: cases in which there is a physical object x that is perceived, but the perception of x is not perceptually mediated by the perception of some *further* physical object, y. Understood as a claim about perceptual mediation, the direct realist will therefore say that, in cases of Φ-terminal perceiving, the perception of x is not perceptually mediated *at all*. For this conception of direct realism, the indirect realist alternative would claim that, in cases of Φ-terminal perceiving, the perception of x *is* perceptually mediated. As the Φ-terminal perception of x could not, by definition, be mediated by perception of some other *physical* object, the indirect theorist would have to claim that it was mediated by perception of something *non*physical as is claimed by certain versions of sense-datum theory. To this extent, indirect realists affirm, while direct realists deny, that perception is always mediated by the perception of something nonphysical.

On this understanding of the direct/indirect distinction, while realist theories that posit nonphysical sense data count as indirect realist, theories such as adverbialism would count as direct. Adverbialists translate sense-datum theorists' talk about sensing or perceiving nonphysical objects in a way that no longer commits us to the existence of nonphysical entities. So where the sense-datum theorist has Pauline's perceiving an apple being mediated by her perceiving (or sensing) a red, round, sense datum, the adverbialist tells us that, when Pauline perceives an apple, she senses redly and roundly—an event that does not intrinsically involve the sensing or perceiving of any *thing* at all. As such a view can agree that, in cases of Φ-terminal perceiving, the perception of x is not mediated by the *perception* of anything at all, adverbialism would therefore count as a form of direct realism.

Some philosophers have suggested that this therefore does not get to the heart of what we are trying to put our finger on when we talk about direct access. As Putnam puts it:

> Sometimes the term [direct] is applied to any position that denies that the objects of 'veridical' perception are sense data. Such a usage makes it much too easy to be a direct realist. All one has to do to be a direct realist (in this sense) … is to say, 'We don't perceive visual experiences, we have them.' A simple linguistic reform, and voila! one is a direct realist.
>
> **Putnam (1994, p. 453)**

Putnam's complaint is thus that, even though conceiving of the distinction between direct and indirect access in terms of perceptual mediation does indeed classify sense-datum theories appropriately, any conception that can be resolved by a simple linguistic reform fails to adequately capture the key question of whether or not our cognitive powers can indeed "reach all the way to the objects themselves."

Foster's second way of drawing the distinction between direct and indirect access cannot be resolved in such a way. This alternative replaces the notion of perceptual mediation with that of *psychological* mediation, on which "S's perceiving of x at t is *psychologically mediated by his being in* Σ if and only if

1. Σ is a psychological state;
2. Σ is not, in itself, x-perceptive (i.e., being in Σ does not, on its own, logically suffice to put one in perceptual contact with x);
3. S's perceiving of x at t breaks down into his being in Σ at t and certain additional facts; and
4. these additional facts do not involve anything further about S's psychological condition at t (anything over and above what is already covered by S's being in Σ)." (Foster, 2000, p. 10).

As any theory that counts as perceptually mediated would also count as psychologically mediated—as the claim that a nonphysical object is perceived (or sensed) would constitute a *theory* of the mediating psychological state Σ—sense-datum theory would count as indirect on both approaches. Note, however, that on *this* way of understanding the distinction between direct and indirect realism, adverbialism would count as *indirect*. As the adverbialist's psychological state of sensing redly and roundly does not intrinsically involve the sensing or perceiving of anything at all, it cannot— by itself—suffice to make it the case that Pauline perceives an apple. And indeed, this is central to the adverbialist's analysis of cases such as dreaming of an apple or hallucinating an apple: Pauline is in Σ—she senses redly and roundly—*in the absence of* an apple. On such a view, for Pauline to actually *perceive* an apple is for her to (1) sense redly and roundly (to be in Σ) *and* (2) for Σ to be caused by an apple in an appropriate manner. Perceiving an apple, as the adverbialist understands it, would therefore count as *psychologically* (if not perceptually) mediated. If psychological mediation is the mark of the indirect, then, adverbialism would count as a version of indirect realism.

In addition to this, some variants of *intentionalist* theories of perception would also count as indirect on this criterion. Intentionalists hold that all perceptual experiences have intentional or representational *contents*. If an intentionalist also holds, along with McGinn (1982) and Davies (1992) that particular objects cannot enter into those contents, then such a version will also probably count as indirect. If we individuate psychological states in such a way that similarities and differences in psychological state track similarities and differences in intentional contents, then the most natural development of such a position would be to hold that, when Pauline perceives an apple, she is in the psychological state, Σ, of perceptually representing *that there is an apple in front of her*. Yet this alone would not suffice to make it the case that Pauline perceives an apple, as she could be in this state when she is under an illusion or suffering from a hallucination. For Pauline to perceive an apple, she would have to *both* be in Σ *and* other things would have to be the case, such as the content of Σ's being true, and for Σ to be caused in an appropriate manner.

Other variants of intentionalism could, however, qualify as direct. Suppose, instead of restricting intentional contents to existentially quantified contents, an intentionalist was to follow Tye (2007) and Schellenberg (2011) in holding that, in veridical cases, perceptual experiences have *singular* contents that are constituted, in part, by the seen objects. Again, if we individuate psychological states in such a way that differences in content yield differences in psychological state, then changes in the object perceived would yield changes in content, which would in turn constitute changes in psychological state. Given this, if a subject S is in a psychological state of perceptually representing particular object x, then this would seem to suffice to make it the case that S perceives x. This version of intentionalism would therefore fail to qualify as psychologically mediated, and hence would qualify as direct.

I want to argue, however, that this way of explaining what direct access consists of also falls prey to something similar to Putnam's complaint. To explain: consider the range of theories that would count as indirect on the psychological mediation criterion. As we have seen, each of these theories will have, at the center of the theory of perception, a mediating psychological state, Σ. As the paradigm examples of perceptual experiences are conscious, there will typically be *something it is like* to perceive. So when we perceive an apple, for example, the color of the apple—its redness, say—is somehow given to us, or made present to us, in the experience's phenomenal character. Following McCulloch (1994, p. 79) we might say that, in such cases, redness is *phenomenologically present*. If—as seems natural—we understand a property being phenomenologically present to a subject to be a psychological fact *about that subject* then, given Foster's fourth condition in his analysis of psychological mediation, the fact that redness is phenomenologically present will be a fact about Σ. Any philosophical analysis of the mediating psychological state will thus, to be complete, have to incorporate an explanation of how being in this state makes it the case that certain properties are phenomenologically present to the subject. So although different theories will offer different explanations of the underlying nature of Σ, for each one we can ask: why does being in Σ make it the case that a particular phenomenal property—in this case, redness—is phenomenologically present?

Importantly, this question cannot be answered simply by saying that redness is phenomenologically present *because* the subject is in Σ; the question we are interested in rather asks *why* being in Σ suffices to make that property phenomenologically present. The answers to this question will differ according to the indirect theory in question. For example, sense-datum theorists would say that redness is phenomenologically present because the sense datum the subject perceives itself instantiates redness. Adverbialists, on the other hand, would say that it is the fact that the subject is sensing *redly* that accounts for the fact that redness is phenomenologically present. And indirect variants of intentionalism would offer different stories still, many of which would appeal to the fact that the subject is in a state, which perceptually represents (in part) the presence of *redness* in the subject's immediate environment.

When these explanations of why being in Σ suffices to make redness phenomenologically present are combined with the fact that—following Foster's (2)—Σ is not, in itself, redness-perceptive, we can see that all of these theories will explain the phenomenological presence of redness *without* requiring redness to be present to the senses. In that light, consider the case in which Pauline does indeed perceive the apple. On these theories, this will be because Pauline is in Σ and certain additional—nonpsychological—facts also obtain. As this is a case of veridical perception then redness will not only be *phenomenologically* present for Pauline but also *perceptually* present—there is a real-world instance of redness that Pauline perceives. So what explains the phenomenological presence of redness in such a case? The fact that Pauline is in Σ. So whatever explanation is provided for why being in Σ suffices to make redness phenomenologically present will also hold for cases in which redness is successfully perceived. Essentially what this shows is that what is going on in Pauline's consciousness is importantly *disconnected* from what is going on in the world around her. Even if the redness of the apple *causes* redness to be phenomenologically present for her, it does not *explain* its phenomenological presence in the deeper sense. This feature of such theories gives another dimension to why it is appropriate to call them indirect.

Let us now turn our attention to those variants of intentionalism that, as we saw, qualified as *direct* on Foster's psychological mediation criteria: what answer do such theories give to the question of why being in a certain psychological state suffices to make a property phenomenologically present? Both Tye and Schellenberg give different answers to this question. Tye develops a view on which "each experience has an SWF [single-when-filled] content into which all the same (non-object involving) properties enter" and "take[s] phenomenal character to be the cluster of properties within the content (singular or gappy)" (Tye, 2007, pp. 608–609). Schellenberg, however, looks not at the properties that the subject is aware of, but at the concepts the subject deploys in becoming aware of those properties. She says "the phenomenology of the experience corresponds one-to-one with the concepts employed in a sensory mode" and that "subjectively indistinguishable experiences share a content element (namely mode of presentation types) that is independent of objects and property-instances" (Schellenberg, 2011, pp. 742–743). What is notable about both of these cases is that, for both Tye and Schellenberg, the aspects of the experience that fix the experience's phenomenal features are *distinct* from those features that are appealed to in the system for psychological state individuation. To the extent that we count experiences of distinct objects—or hallucinations of those objects—as different psychological states, it is because we appeal to the singular aspects of the content in claiming that the contents, and hence psychological states, are different; yet it is precisely these aspects of the psychological state that are then disregarded in the explanations of how the phenomenal aspects of the experience are fixed.

This suggests that Foster's move from perceptual to psychological mediation has not adequately resolved Putnam's original concern. Putnam objected to drawing the direct/indirect distinction in such a way that a simple linguistic choice could make the difference as to whether a theory provided us with direct or indirect access to mind-independent reality: the difference between direct and indirect access should be more philosophically substantive than *that*. What these considerations show is that the psychological mediation definition has a similar problem: all one has to do to be a direct realist (in *this* sense) is to say, "We do not individuate psychological states by the common content types that fix phenomenal character, but by the singular content tokens that these types yield." A simple reform of psychological methodology, and *voila!* one is a direct realist.[1]

To approach this concern in another way, consider why we find it worth distinguishing between direct and indirect access in the first place, and why understanding this distinction in terms of perceptual mediation has prima facie plausibility. Suppose that the sense-datum theory were true, and that all perceptual experience—veridical and hallucinatory—proceeded via awareness of nonphysical sense data. On such a view, when Pauline perceives an apple, she perceives the apple *in virtue of* perceiving, or sensing, a nonphysical object. But as she could have had an experience *just like this* in the absence of an apple, then things would be just like this—in the realm of Pauline's subjectivity—even if there were no apple in this world. This raises the "veil of perception" concern: if the object we are directly aware of is the same in both cases (the apple-shaped and colored sense datum), then in what sense does having direct access to this object really give us indirect access to an object of some other kind? These considerations start to make us question whether indirect access to the apple really counts as *access* at all. Sense data seem problematic because they can seem to *block* our awareness from reaching all the way to the apple, which is why a theory that does not posit intermediate *objects*—a theory that rejects perceptual mediation—can seem to be what is required to calm the waters. As Putnam puts it, the underlying concern with indirect access is really "the idea that there has to be an interface between our cognitive powers and the external world – or, to put the same point differently, the idea that our cognitive powers cannot reach all the way to the objects themselves" (Putnam, 1994, p. 453). But Putnam's complaint is that this concern should not be able to be adequately resolved by a simple linguistic reform. But then—regardless of the precise account of how phenomenal character is fixed—so long as it is the case that the psychological features that fix the phenomenal character of Pauline's experience are independent of whether or not there is an apple

---

[1] Tyler Burge (2005) argues that it should be left to perceptual psychology to set the appropriate individuative criteria for psychological states. This would suggests that there is in fact a "right answer" as to how we should individuate perceptual states, and hence—contrary to the above—that we cannot just choose a different methodology. In response to Burge, however, John McDowell (2010) contends that the philosophy and psychology of perception are engaged in different explanatory projects, and that what counts as appropriate individuative criteria for perceptual psychology should not be assumed to carry over to more traditionally philosophical projects. To this extent, then, there is still scope for philosophers to prefer different individuative practices for different enterprises, and the concern stands that the decision as to how to individuate perceptual states should not be the sole determinant of whether that theory provides direct, or merely indirect, access to mind-independent objects.

in Pauline's immediate environment, the concern remains: things would be just like this—in the realm of Pauline's subjectivity—even if there were no apple in this world. The move to understanding the distinction between direct and indirect realism in terms of psychological mediation has not got to the heart of the issue.

Instead, I suggest that a better way to draw the distinction between direct and indirect perception is in terms of *phenomenal mediation*. Adapting Foster's conditions for perception to count as psychologically mediated, we might define this notion as follows:

S's perceiving of x at t is phenomenally mediated by phenomenal character ψ *if and only if*

1. *ψ is a phenomenal character;*
2. *ψ is not, in itself, x-perceptive; and*
3. *S's perceiving of x at t breaks down into his being the subject of ψ at t and certain additional facts;*[2]

What would it be for a phenomenal character ψ to be x-perceptive? Well, thinking back to our discussion of psychological mediation, if ψ is x-perceptive, then being the subject of ψ would suffice for you to be in perceptual contact with x. But what does this notion of "perceptual contact" really mean? Our discussions so far suggest that it is for x (and its properties) to be *phenomenologically* present to the subject of ψ or, alternatively, for ψ to be x-*involving*. If the phenomenal character of Pauline's apple experience were apple *involving* in this way, then if the apple (or any of its properties) were different, or absent, then things would be *different* for Pauline in the realm of her subjectivity.[3]

If we define indirect access as access that is *phenomenally* mediated in this way, then even singular versions of intentionalism would—so long as the explanation of why being in a certain psychological state suffices to make a property phenomenologically present appeals to features of the psychological state common to veridical and nonveridical cases—qualify as indirect. In this way, we can define a notion of direct access that clearly shows how, in

---

[2] Note that there is not a counterpart of Foster's (4) for phenomenal mediation. This is because the additional facts that need to be added to the bare fact of S's being the subject of ψ could include additional facts about S's psychological condition at t, such as the fact that the mental state to which ψ attaches has a singular content of a certain kind.

[3] This is not to say that Pauline would be guaranteed to *notice* any of these potential differences. There are many reasons why Pauline may fail to be aware of relevant differences, ranging from her basic recognitional abilities to the allocation of her attention. I will discuss these issues in more detail in Section 2 below.

cases of direct access, our cognitive powers "reach all the way to the objects themselves": S's perceiving of x at t would count as giving S direct access to x if and only if S enjoyed a phenomenal character that was x-involving, and thus made x (and its properties) *phenomenologically present* to S.[4]

2. PART II: DISJUNCTIVISM AND DIRECT REALISM

The first part of this paper argued that a third way to understand the notion of indirect perception—in terms of the presence of phenomenal mediation—best captures the underlying motivation for distinguishing between direct and indirect perception in the first place. In the remainder of the paper, I shall now show that direct perception—thus understood—not only entails disjunctivism but also a specific form of disjunctivism.

The thread that holds different disjunctive theories together is the underlying claim that the mental states involved in a veridical perceptual experience differ from those involved in a "bad case" experience of hallucination, even in those cases in which the two experiences are indistinguishable for their subject.[5] But of course—as we saw above when we discussed different approaches to the individuation of psychological states—our criteria for determining whether two states count as the same or different can differ. For example, we might develop an epistemological disjunctivism by claiming that perceptual and hallucinatory states count as different so long as they differ in their status as perceptual evidence, regardless of any other similarities they might share. Alternatively, the metaphysical disjunctivist will hold that perceptual and hallucinatory states count as different so long as they have different constituents—perhaps in virtue of involving singular contents. As we saw above, however, two mental states could have different

---

[4] It may be argued that phenomenal mediation is too strong for (mere) direct realism and should instead be viewed as criteria for *naïve* realism. On such a view, a theory would count as a version of direct realism so long as the kind of experience you have when you see an object could not have occurred in the absence of that object, and a version of naïve realism, so long as the conscious character of the experience you have when you see an object could not have occurred in the absence of that object. If somebody wants to use the terms in this way, then I have no objection: what I would suggest, though, is that—on this way of naming theories—our real interest would be in naïve, rather than direct, realism.

[5] Again, Burge (2005) insists that the mental states that are of interest to the philosopher *just are* the psychological states that are of interest to the psychologist, and hence that, in making this claim, disjunctivism runs counter to the claims of vision science. For the reasons given by McDowell (2010), however, the disjunctivist will deny this, holding instead that disjunctivism about the mental states involved in perception is compatible with the presence of common psychological states, as understood by visual psychology. To try and keep this clear, I talk about mental states, rather than psychological states, when discussing disjunctivism.

constituents—and hence count as a version of disjunctivism on this criteria—even while the aspects of experience that fixed the experience's phenomenal character were common to perceptual and hallucinatory cases. The only version of disjunctivism that will guarantee a theory provides for direct access to mind-independent reality is thus a *phenomenal* disjunctivism. This approach effectively individuates mental states by their phenomenal character—so two mental states count as different if and only if they differ in their phenomenal character.[6] Only if a theory of perception is phenomenally disjunctive will it be able to guarantee that the phenomenal character involved in a case of veridical perception would suffice for the subject to be in perceptual contact with the world. On the phenomenal mediation understanding of direct realism, then, a direct realist will not only have to be a disjunctivist but also a phenomenal disjunctivist. But the constraints do not stop there. For as I shall now argue, phenomenal disjunctivism requires negative disjunctivism.

To see why, note that the core *commitment* of the phenomenal disjunctivist is that veridical perceptions and hallucinations have different phenomenology, or phenomenal character, and the core *constraint* of the theory is that such experiences can, nonetheless, be indiscriminable from one another. So suppose the phenomenal disjunctivist offers the kind of relationalist or naïve realist theory of veridical perceptual phenomenology that would logically suffice for the subject of that phenomenology to be in perceptual contact with the world. What can the phenomenal disjunctivist then say about the phenomenology of the indiscriminable hallucination? For obvious reasons, the theory cannot be the same as it is for the veridical case, so what are the phenomenal disjunctivist's options here?

The most natural first suggestion would be to provide a positive theory of the phenomenology of hallucination that differed from that provided in the veridical case. Indeed, we might pick any of the theories of perception that we have thus far considered—sense-datum theories, adverbialism, intentionalism—and retool it as a theory of the phenomenology *of*

---

[6] I say "effectively" because it is not impossible to imagine a theory that individuated mental states in such a way—by narrow functional role, say—that veridical perceptions and their indiscriminable hallucinations qualified as the same mental state, while nonetheless offering a theory of phenomenal character that allowed the same mental state to have different phenomenal character in different circumstances. Unusual as such a theory would be, one might argue that it would not qualify as a version of disjunctivism, in as much as there is a common mental state to indiscriminable cases of perception and hallucination. While that may be the case, such a theory would nonetheless seem to qualify as disjunctivism *about phenomenology*, inasmuch as the indiscriminable cases of perception and hallucination do not have phenomenology or phenomenal character in common.

the hallucinatory case alone.[7] Suppose, for the sake of argument, we pick the sense-datum theory (although nothing of substance hangs on this choice) and hold that, in cases of hallucination, we perceive (or sense) a nonphysical object that is indiscriminable from the *physical* object that is seen in the associated veridical case. This in turn raises the question of: *why* do we perceive (or sense) a nonphysical object in such a case? Given what we know about the causal etiology of states such as hallucinations and dreams, it appears that they can be the result of neural activity alone. So suppose we develop the theory as follows: in cases of hallucination, we sense a sense datum *because* neural activity of the right kind takes place. So regardless of the particular theory we choose, the underlying point is that the neural activity alone must suffice for an experience—however understood—that is indiscriminable from a veridical perception.

With the theory developed in this way, we can now ask whether neural activity of this kind would *also* take place in *veridical* cases. At this point, the positive phenomenal disjunctivist seems to have three choices: (1) to deny that the relevant neural activity could occur in veridical cases; (2) to allow that the relevant neural activity could also occur in veridical cases but insist that, in such cases, the subject would not suffice for an indiscriminable experience; (3) to allow that the relevant neural activity could also occur in veridical cases and to accept that, in such cases, it would also suffice for an indiscriminable experience. Response (1) is possible, but note that it must be more extensive than the simple claim that the neural activity will differ in cases of hallucination and veridical perception. To endorse (1), we would have to claim that the neural activity that suffices for the indiscriminable experience does not even occur *as a constituent of* the overall neural activity that takes place in perceptual cases. This would seem to make the overall project a hostage to empirical fortune, as well as to conflict with philosophical intuitions about the effects of neural replication. Response (2) also faces significant challenges. As Robinson wonders, "if the mechanism or brain state is a sufficient causal condition for the production of [an indiscriminable experience] when the [objects] are not there, why is it not so sufficient when they are present? Does the brain state mysteriously know how it is being produced... or does the [object],

---

[7] Indeed, Benj Hellie (2013) has recently argued that we need not pick just one of these theories and that, by adopting such a "multidisjunctive" conception of hallucination, we can avoid the argument I am about to present. This is an intriguing suggestion, but it looks poorly motivated without a reason to think that there might be different positive theories of hallucination that apply to different subjects.

when present, inhibit the production of [an indiscriminable experience] by some sort of action at a distance?" (Robinson, 1994, pp. 153–154). This just looks implausible: if the neural activity suffices for the subject to have an experience that is indiscriminable from a veridical experience in the *absence* of an appropriate object, surely it will also be sufficient when the object is there. That seems to leave the positive phenomenal disjunctivist with response (3).

According to this response, when the same neural activity that occurs during a hallucination takes place in a case of veridical perception, it would suffice for the subject to have an experience that is indiscriminable from a veridical experience. But this is in tension with the (phenomenal mediation) direct realist's endorsement of the kind of relationalist or naïve realist theory of veridical perceptual phenomenology that would logically suffice for the subject of that phenomenology to be in perceptual contact with the world. As we have seen, all this talk of phenomenology or phenomenal character is supposed to capture what it is like for the subject, or how things are for the subject from their particular conscious perspective. So when Pauline perceives an apple, what it is like, for Pauline, is like a particular apple being phenomenologically present to her. The relationalist will want to claim that the reason it is like this for Pauline is because the apple *really is* present in the phenomenology of her experience. But if the phenomenal disjunctivist has endorsed response (3), they already have an explanation of why it is like this for Pauline—it is like this for Pauline because of the neural activity she is undergoing. How it is from the subject's perspective has already been accounted for by the experience that is produced by the neural activity alone. At best this has the consequence that what is like for perceiving subjects is systematically overdetermined; more plausibly, it provides us with reasons to think that what it is like to perceive veridically is not really x-involving after all. So regardless of what particular approach to hallucination is adopted, the worry is that as soon as the phenomenal direct realist gives a substantive theory of the phenomenal aspects of hallucination, they will have thereby given an account that can be extended to explain the conscious character of veridical perception too. The supposedly x-involving features of veridical perceptual phenomenology are not needed to explain what it is like for Pauline—they have been "screened off" from playing an important explanatory role.

What we therefore find is that the positive disjunctivist view is threatened by a "veil" of phenomenology, much like indirect realist theories are threatened by a veil of perception. In the latter case, the worry is that, if a theory insists that we are aware of mind-dependent *objects* in perception, then these objects will really serve to *block* us from being aware of the mind-*independent* objects in the external world. In the present case, the concern is rather that, if the positive disjunctivist offers a positive account of hallucinatory phenomenology that is generated by neural activity alone, then this phenomenology will also be present in veridical cases and will thus *block* the purported apple-involving phenomenology from playing a role in what it is like from the subject's perspective.

In response to this "screening off" worry, M.G.F. Martin argues that common properties with "inherited or dependent explanatory potential offer us exceptions to the general model of common properties screening off special ones" (2004, p. 70). To explain, consider an unattended bag in an airport. When an object has this property, it causes a security alert. Why? Because although objects with this property are usually harmless, this is not always the case: sometimes they contain a bomb. In this light, consider Bag A, which is a harmless piece of mislaid luggage, and Bag B, which contains a bomb. Both Bag A and Bag B have the property of being an unattended bag in an airport, while Bag B also has the property of being a bomb in an airport. As both bags have the property of being an unattended bag in an airport, they both cause a security alert. Now consider Bag B. Does the property it shares with Bag A—that of being an unattended bag in an airport—screen off the noncommon property of being a bomb in an airport from being explanatory? Does it mean that Bag B's being a bomb in an airport is irrelevant in explaining why a security alert occurred? Surely not. The only reason the common property of being an unattended bag in an airport has the explanatory role it does in the first place is because, sometimes, this property is correlated with the property that we are really interested in: the property of being a bomb in an airport. In such a case, the explanatory potential of the common property (of being an unattended bag in airport) is "inherited from" or "dependent on" the explanatory potential of the special property of being a bomb in an airport. Martin then puts this insight into work as follows. He accepts that both a veridical perception of a certain kind and an indiscriminable hallucination have a common property: that of being indiscriminable from a veridical perception of that kind (as the veridical perception will of course be indiscriminable from itself). Yet, just as in the bag case, he suggests that whatever explanatory potential this common property has is entirely inherited from the special (naïve realist) property possessed by the associated veridical experience alone.

Why did James shriek like that? He was in a situation indiscriminable from the veridical perception of a spider. Given James's fear of spiders, when confronted with one he is liable so to react; and with no detectable difference between this situation and such a perception, it must seem to him as if a spider is there, so he reacts in the same way.

Martin (2004, p. 68)

Martin thus concludes that to avoid the screening off worry, the disjunctivist should characterize the hallucinatory state purely negatively: when it comes to a mental characterization of the hallucinatory experience, nothing more can be said than the relational and epistemological claim that it is indiscriminable from the perception (2004, p. 72) With this kind of negative, epistemic analysis of hallucination, Martin suggests we can avoid the claim that the naïve realist aspects of a veridical experience will be screened off from explaining what it is like from the subject's perspective. Instead of claiming that veridical perceptions and their associated hallucinations are indiscriminable because they have a common property that accounts for the fact that they both shape the contours of the subject's conscious experiences in the same way, Martin contends that veridical perceptions shape the contours of the subject's conscious experience in a particular way because they have a special naïve realist property, and that hallucinations can only be said to shape them in the same way inasmuch as they have the (common) property of being indiscriminable from veridical experiences that have this special property.

Importantly, while taking this line does require the phenomenal disjunctivist to resist giving a positive account of the phenomenology of hallucination, this does not amount to denying that hallucinations have phenomenology at all (as I explain in Fish, 2013). As we have seen, when we talk about phenomenology, we are intending to talk about how things are from the subject's perspective or point of view. Veridical, visual perceptual experiences contribute to what it is like from the subject's perspective: in having such experiences, the subject's perspective will embody an openness to or awareness of aspects of its environment. When you have a subject that is open to its environment in this kind of way, a whole array of different mental states can contribute, in different ways, to what it is like *for that subject*. Hallucinations, in particular—as states that are indiscriminable from a veridical perception of a certain kind—make it, *for the subject*, just like they are having a certain kind of veridical perception. How do they do this? Because the subject of such states *takes themselves to be having a veridical perception of a certain kind* and *there is something it is like to have that veridical perception*. It is because veridical perceptual states have x-perceptive phenomenal character that there is something it is like to have a veridical perception and it is only because there is something it is like to have a veridical perception that there is something it is like to *mistakenly take oneself* to have a veridical perception. So the explanation of the phenomenology of hallucination *requires* both that veridical perceptions will have a phenomenology and that this phenomenology must be explained in a different way to that of hallucination. What is more, it gives an intuitive account of what it is like for the hallucinating subject: where what it is like to perceive is determined by the elements of the environment the subject is open to in experience, what it is like to hallucinate is determined by the kind of openness one mistakenly takes oneself to be enjoying, Thus whatever hallucinations contribute to what it is like from the perspective of a conscious subject, both the very fact that they contribute at all, as well as the particular contribution they make, is entirely parasitic on the contribution made by veridical experiences.

REFERENCES

Bennett, J., 1971. Locke, Berkeley, Hume: Central Themes. Oxford University Press, New York.
Burge, T., 2005. Disjunctivism and perceptual psychology. Philos. Top. 33, 1–78.
Davies, M., 1992. Perceptual content and local supervenience. Proc. Aristot. Soc. 92, 21–46.
Fish, W., 2013. Perception, hallucination, and illusion: reply to my critics. Philos. Stud. 163, 57–66.
Foster, J., 2000. The Nature of Perception. Oxford University Press, Oxford.
Hellie, B., 2013. The multidisjunctive conception of hallucination. In: Macpherson, F., Platchias, D. (Eds.), Hallucination. The MIT Press, Cambridge, MA, pp. 221–254.
Locke, J., 1961. In: Yolton, J. (Ed.), An Essay Concerning Human Understanding. Everyman's Library, London and New York.
Martin, M.G.F., 2004. "The Limits of Self-Awareness." Philosophical Studies 120, 37–89.
McCulloch, G., 1994. Using Sartre: An Analytical Introduction to Early Sartrean Themes. Routledge, London.
McDowell, J., 2010. Tyler Burge on disjunctivism. Philos. Explor. 13, 243–255.
McGinn, C., 1982. The Character of Mind. Oxford University Press, Oxford.
Putnam, H., 1994. Sense, nonsense and the senses: an inquiry into the powers of the human mind. J. Phil. 91 (9), 445–517.
Robinson, H., 1994. Perception. Routledge, London.
Schellenberg, S., 2011. Perceptual content defended. Noûs 45, 714–750.
Tye, M., 2007. Intentionalism and the argument from no common content. Philos. Perspect. 21, 589–613.

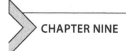

CHAPTER NINE

Perceptual Realism's Fundamental Forms

Pierre Le Morvan

Department of Philosophy, Religion, and Classical Studies, The College of New Jersey, Ewing, NJ, United States

> Naïve (or spontaneous) *realism holds that the world is just as we see it,* i.e., *that we know it directly through our senses.*
>
> *Mario Bunge (1977, p. 262)*

> *[T]he question of whether or not naïve realism (or something like it) is true is the central problem in the philosophy of perception.*
>
> *Matthew Nudds (2009, p. 334n1)*

1. INTRODUCTION

The philosophy of perception has undergone a historic shift since the widespread abandonment of the sense-datum theory in the 1950s, whereas the rejection of Perceptual Realism prevailed from at least the 17th century until then; since then Perceptual Realism has made a remarkable comeback. But what exactly is Perceptual Realism? The purpose of this chapter is to delineate its fundamental forms.

To begin we may note that Perceptual Realism holds in essence that perception-independent physical objects are what perceivers perceive. It should be borne in mind that "object" is meant here to include not only things (such as tables and gables) but also events (such as barking beagles or lightning flashes), substances (such as water or gold), or stuffs (such as flour or sand). An important form of Perceptual Realism is Direct Realism, and here a terminological matter merits our attention.

2. DIRECT REALISM DISTINGUISHED FROM NAÏVE REALISM

The terms "Direct Realism" and "Naïve Realism" (or more rarely "Naïf Realism") are often used interchangeably in the literature—even by many of those who consider themselves perceptual realists (For examples, see Appendix A.). But doing so proves regrettable for three main reasons.

Direct versus Indirect Realism
ISBN 978-0-12-812141-2
https://doi.org/10.1016/B978-0-12-812141-2.00009-X

The first is that "naïve" is typically used in a way that connotes a lack of experience, or judgment, or wisdom; to be naïve is thus to be credulous or gullible as indicated OED's definition 1 of "naïve." It's no surprise then that detractors of Direct Realism—who described it as a commonsense or folk view incapable of withstanding philosophical scrutiny—pejoratively labeled it as "Naïve Realism" as did Paulsen and Thilly (1895, p. 334) and Price (1932, p. 27) or as "Naïf Realism" as did Broad (1914, p. 1). Far from being a position that only the gullible or credulous could accept, however, Direct Realism can actually be quite a sophisticated position, and hence to label it as "Naïve" or "Naïf" from the get-go risks mischaracterizing it with misleading connotations.

The second reason is that some varieties of Direct Realism *are*, as we shall see, aptly described as naïve, and so it's best to reserve the moniker "Naïve Realism" for *them* and not for Direct Realism as a genus more broadly. This will help us to avoid the error of thinking that the latter has been refuted just because one or more naïve versions of it have, and to recognize that it is not just opponents of Direct Realism who reject naïve versions of it, but that proponents of it can do so as well, a fact obscured by using "Naïve Realism" and "Direct Realism" interchangeably.

A third reason is that, given the connotations noted above, "Naïve Realism" is sometimes taken simply as a name for an error. As a case in point, Satel and Lilienfeld (2013, p. xi) write: "Plausibly, the survival advantage of vision gave rise to our reflective bias for believing that the world is as we perceive it to be, an error that psychologists and philosophers call naïve realism. This misplaced faith in the trustworthiness of our perceptions is the wellspring of two of history's most famously misguided theories: that the world is flat and that the sun revolves around the earth." While Satel and Lillienfeld overgeneralize particularly about how philosophers use the term "Naïve Realism," at least some philosophers and psychologists do use the term in this way to designate what they take to be an error. It begs the question against Direct Realism to assume that the only version of it is an error.

3. DIRECT REALISM, IDEALISM, AND PHENOMENALISM

What then is Direct Realism? In the most basic sense, it's a form of Perceptual Realism because it takes perception-independent physical objects to be what perceivers perceive, and it's called *direct* because it denies that perceiving them requires a logically prior awareness of an objectified appearance (such as a sense datum, Cartesian–Lockean idea, quality instance, species, or what have you) mediating between perceivers and the perceived. Direct Realism thus proves logically incompatible with rival views of the ontology of perception such as Indirect Realism and forms of Perceptual Anti-Realism such as Idealism and Phenomenalism.

Indirect Realism, like Direct Realism, is also (as you would expect) a form of Perceptual Realism in taking putatively perception-independent physical things to be objects of perception. Unlike Direct Realism, however, Indirect Realism takes perception to be indirect in requiring a logically prior awareness of an objectified appearance that mediates between perceivers and the perceived. Thus, while we do perceive physical objects according to Indirect Realism, we do so only indirectly and in virtue of a prior awareness of objectified appearances mediating between us and physical things. Historically, Descartes and Locke were paradigmatic Indirect Realists.

In common with Indirect Realism, Perceptual Anti-Realism denies that perception is an immediate or direct awareness of perception-independent physical objects, but it goes further in taking perception to be an awareness of perception-dependent objects. Perceptual Anti-Realism comes in two principal forms: Idealism and Phenomenalism. Whereas Idealism take the existence of the perceived to be dependent on its being perceived (*esse est percipi*), Phenomenalism takes the existence of the perceived to be dependent on the possibility of its being perceived (*esse est posse percipi*). Historically, Berkeley was a paradigmatic Idealist, whereas J.S. Mill was a paradigmatic Phenomenalist.

4. FUNDAMENTAL FORMS OF DIRECT REALISM

Having contrasted Direct Realism with Indirect Realism and with Idealism and Phenomenalism, the two principal forms of Perceptual Anti-Realism, let us distinguish between fundamental forms of Direct Realism. Let us begin with what we may call *Ur-Direct Realism*.

4.1 Ur-Direct Realism

Ur-Direct Realism is the common root of all forms of Direct Realism and is nothing more than the thesis that we perceive physical objects without a logically prior awareness of an objectified appearance. Notice that this negational thesis concerns what perception of physical objects does *not* involve: an objectified appearance. Ur-Direct Realism divides into two main forms that we may call *Reducibilist* and *Irreducibilist*, respectively.

4.2 Reducibilist Direct Realism

Reducibilist forms of Direct Realism accept Ur-Direct Realism but conceive of the relation of phenomenal appearance between perceived and perceiver as reducible to something more ontologically fundamental. Adverbialism—which takes perceptual experience to be an essentially objectless way of sensing or being appeared to, a state or event in the perceiver whereby one or more sensory properties are instantiated—is a primary form of Reducibilist Direct Realism. Intentionalism—which takes phenomenal appearance in perceptual experience to consist in an intentional relation between perceived and perceiver—is another form of Reducibilist Direct Realism only if it is distinct from Adverbialism. See Le Morvan (2008) for a discussion of why important forms of Intentionalism turn out to be forms of Adverbialism.

4.3 Irreducibilist Direct Realism

Irreducibilist forms of Direct Realism accept Ur-Direct Realism but go further in conceiving of phenomenal appearance in perceptual experience as an irreducible relation of phenomenal appearing between perceived and perceiver. That is, both perceived and perceiver are relata of this appearing relation—a relation not reducible to anything more ontologically fundamental—and the perceived is a constituent of perception. Irreducibilist Direct Realism comes in two main forms that we may call *Moderate* and *Naïve*, respectively. To see how they differ, consider the difference between *objectual* and *qualitative* veridicality of perceptual experience and the concomitant notion of *appearance-reality gaps*.

A perceptual experience is *objectually veridical* only if at least one physical object *o* phenomenally appears to a percipient and so is a relatum and constituent of the experience. (Note that this physical object need not be—though it typically is—external to the percipient's body. We will see why in due course.) A perceptual experience is *qualitatively veridical* only if at least one physical object *o* phenomenally appears to the percipient as it is; that is, *o* not only phenomenally appears *F* to the percipient but also is *F*, where *F* is some property or relation.

Appearance-reality gaps are divergences between how an object phenomenally appears to a perceiver and how it really is. They can be understood as cases where a perceptual experience is *objectually* veridical (such that a physical object *o* phenomenally appears to a percipient) without being *qualitatively* veridical (such that *o* phenomenally appears *F* to the percipient without being *F*). Henceforth, when I write "appearance-reality gap" I mean it in this sense. Perceptual illusions (*e.g.*, putatively straight sticks appearing bent when partially submerged in water, putatively white objects appearing red when bathed in red light, and so on) provide stock examples of appearance-reality gaps. Hallucinations may be another depending on how they are conceptualized. If hallucinations, however, are construed as perceptual experiences that are not objectually veridical, there is no appearance-reality gap in the way it is understood here, for hallucination so construed would not present anything real since it fails to be objectually veridical.

Moderate and Naïve Forms of Irreducibilist Direct Realism are in agreement that a perceptual experience's being objectually veridical is a necessary condition for it to count as a perception, and its being qualitatively veridical is a sufficient condition therefor. They differ, however, on their admittance of appearance-reality gaps: Moderate Irreducibilist Direct Realism admits them, while Naïve Irreducibilist Direct Realism does not. A view known as the theory of appearing is a form of the former but not the latter. (I defend this view in a work in progress titled *Appearance and Experience: From Realism and Back Again*. See also Alston, 1999).

Let us look next more closely at Naïve Irreducibilist Direct Realism by considering its global and local forms.

4.4 Global and Local Naïve Irreducibilist Direct Realisms

Global Naïve Realism—short for Global Naïve Irreducibilist Direct Realism—brooks no appearance-reality gaps, maintaining in effect that objectual and qualitative veridicality of perceptual experience always covary. By contrast, Local Naïve Realisms (short for Local Naïve Irreducibilist Direct Realisms) deny some, but not all, appearance-reality gaps and can be distinguished by their respective *perceptual naïveté*, the denial of a kind of appearance-reality gap. Thus, while accepting Global Naïve Realism entails accepting all Local Naïve Realisms, accepting some Local Naïve Realism does not by itself entail accepting Global Naïve Realism or another Local Naïve Realism.

At least six kinds of such naïveté may be distinguished: *temporal, chromatic, formal, motional, quantitative*, and *relational*.

To be *temporally naïve* is to think that when we see (or visually perceive) something, it phenomenally appears to us as it is *now* (namely, instantaneously or with temporal immediacy).

To be *chromatically naïve* is to think that when we see something, it phenomenally appears to us exactly as it is *in terms of its color(s)*; that is, the perceived has the color(s) it appears to have—at least for normal percipients in normal conditions, however, these are specified.

To be *formally naïve* is to think that when we see something, it phenomenally appears to us exactly as it is *in terms of its shape(s) or structure(s)*; in other words, that the perceived has the shape(s) or structure(s) it appears to have.

To be *quantitatively* naïve is to think that when we see something, it phenomenally appears to us exactly as it is *in terms of its quantity.*

To be *motionally naïve* is to think that when we see something, it phenomenally appears to us exactly as it is *in terms of its motion.*

To be *relationally naïve* is to think that when we see something, it phenomenally appears to us exactly as it is *in terms of its relations.*

Having distinguished Global Naïve Realism from Local Naïve Realism and six forms of the latter, it's worth noting that while each entails Direct Realism, Direct Realism does not entail any of them, for one can be a Moderate Direct Realist and reject each of these forms of perceptual naïveté. Thus, even if an argument succeeds in refuting some form of Naïve Direct Realism, it does not follow that Direct Realism itself has been refuted.

5. DOES ANYONE SUBSCRIBE TO GLOBAL OR LOCAL NAÏVE REALISM?

I distinguished earlier between Direct Realism and Naïve Realism, arguing in effect for the wisdom of not using terms for them interchangeably. Given the distinctions drawn above between kinds of Naïve Realism, a question worth asking is whether anyone actually subscribes to Naïve Realism. Let me distinguish between two ways of taking this question. The first concerns whether, as a matter of psychology, we humans tend to unreflectingly subscribe to (some form of) such realism. The second concerns whether, as a matter of philosophy, any philosophers subscribe on reflection to some form of it.

As to the first question, the answer seems to be clearly yes. As psychologists Pronin et al. (2004) note:

> The core of naïve realism is the conviction that one perceives objects and events 'as they are' (…) This conviction is inescapable and deep, and it governs our day-to-day functioning despite what we may know about the constructive nature of perception. Thus, even when we have learned that the colors and objects we perceive reflect the interaction between a world of molecules and energy sources and our particular human sensory processes, we continue to respond to the relevant stimuli in accord with our naive conviction about objective reality. We accept the word of scientists that this world is perceived very differently by other creatures—that the sounds, sights, and smells they experience may scarcely resemble our own. But we tend to regard those creatures as having an altered perspective on the objective properties of the reality we perceive, rather than vice versa (p. 783).

Pronin et al. (2004) also note that we expect other reasonable and attentive people to perceive the same reality we do, and, when others disagree with us, we tend to deem our own views as dictated by objective reality and any disagreement as the result of some idiosyncrasy on the part of disagreers.

As for the second question, the answer is less obvious. To see why, let us consider some recent representative statements of what Naïve Realism supposedly amounts to—statements given by three philosophers in important recent works in defense of what they themselves label as "Naïve Realism."

Campbell (2002) defends what he calls "the Relational View," which he characterizes as a form of Naïve Realism (p. 118). On this view, "the phenomenal character of your experience, as you look around the room, is constituted by the actual layout of the room itself: which particular objects are there, their intrinsic properties, such as colour and shape, and how they are arranged in relation to one another and to you" (p. 116). As far as *this* statement goes, Campbell seems to be articulating a form of Naïve Realism, even of Global Naïve Realism, as I use these terms; however, he later cautions that the Relational View "is consistent with saying that only certain of the characteristics of the objects one is seeing constitute one's experience of them" (p. 120), and that things can also appear other than they are such as things appearing in a yellow cast to the jaundiced (p. 118). So Campbell clearly does not subscribe to Global Naïve Realism; as for Local Naïve Realisms, he appears to not subscribe to Chromatic Naïve Realism insofar as he holds that objects may appear other than they are in terms of their color, and it's an open question the extent to which he subscribes to the other Local Naïve Realisms.

According to Martin (2004, p. 39), the Naïve Realist claims that our sense experience of the world is, at least in part, non-representational. Some of the objects of perception – the concrete individuals, their properties, the events these partake in – are constituents of the experience. No experience like this, no experience of fundamentally the same kind, could have occurred had no appropriate candidate for awareness existed. In this, sense perception contrasts with imagining and thought. For one can certainly imagine objects in their absence, so the mind's direction on an object does not require that it actually exist when one imagines. The same is true, arguably, of thought – we think of objects which in fact do not exist as well as thinking of the existent.

Once again, as far as *this* statement goes, Martin also seems to be articulating a form of Naïve Realism, even of Global Naïve Realism, as I understand these terms; however, we later find him retreating to the more restricted thesis that *in nonhallucinatory, nonillusory cases* external objects and their features "shape the contours of the subject's conscious experience"

(p. 64). Martin thus clearly does not subscribe to Global Naïve Realism. But as to the extent to which he subscribes to other Local Naïve Realisms, we are left with an open question.

Fish (2009, p. 6) echoes Martin in saying that Naïve Realism is the view that external objects and their properties shape the contours of the subject's conscious experience "by actually *being* the contours of the subject's conscious experience." On the face of it, with this statement Fish too seems to be articulating a form of Naïve Realism, even of Global Naïve Realism as I understand these terms. According to Fish (2010, p. 96), the Naïve Realist "holds that, whenever we have a case of conscious perception, there is something the subject is aware of and that bears the properties that characterize what it is like for the subject...and these objects of awareness are actually the mind-independent objects that inhabit the world." Since Fish recognizes, however, the occurrence of illusions and hallucinations, he clearly does not subscribe to Global Naïve Realism; as to the extent of the Local Naïve Realisms he subscribes to, we are yet again left with an open question. Fish (2009) does defend a kind of Chromatic Realism according to which "the specific color a particular exhibits on any given occasion depends not only upon its intrinsic surface properties, but also on facts about its 'setting'—facts about the illuminant and the object's surround" (p. 153). He adds that although "these color-determining aspects are not intrinsic aspects of the particular itself, they are still aspects of the objective physical world" and claims that "a realist about color—which, of course, the naïve realist must be—might conceivably attempt to accommodate these factors in a theory of color" (p. 153) Notice here the way he ties Naïve Realism to Chromatic Realism.

These three notable philosophers, self-described Naïve Realists, thus give us a characterization of Naïve Realism that we may encapsulate as holding that, in nonillusory, nonhallucinatory perceptual experience, physical objects appear to us as they are and are constituents of that experience. While clearly not committed to Global Naïve Realism, this characterization leaves regrettably underspecified the extent of its commitment to Local Naïve Realisms. I think that this underspecification in characterizations of Naïve Realism is at least partly a result of a failure to explicitly distinguish between objectual and qualitative veridicality and between various kinds of Local Naïve Realisms and their respective perceptual naïveté. (For some additional examples of this underspecification, see Appendix B.)

6. CONCLUSION

We have seen in this chapter the fundamental forms that Perceptual Realism can take. Direct Realism has been *deconflated* from Naïve Realism, and Moderate Direct Realism has been distinguished from global and local Forms of Naïve Realism. In light of these distinctions, both defenders and rejecting of Perpetual Realism would be wise to clearly specify the kind of Perceptual Realism they are supporting or rejecting.

APPENDIX A

Representative examples of the tendency to treat the terms "Direct Realism" and "Naïve Realism" interchangeably include the following:

Common Sense Philosophy reappeared in the twentieth century in theories of direct or naïve realism (we directly perceive objects, not ideas or sense or sense data.

Beck (1966, p. 132)

Whereas direct (or naïve) realists hold that the immediate objects of phenomenal awareness are physical objects or their surfaces, representational (or Lockean-style indirect) realists hold that the immediate objects of perception are phenomenal. I call it 'direct realism,' but it is also often called 'naïve realism,' a name which reflects both its appeal to common sense and the assessment of many philosophers that it is open to clear and decisive objections.

Huemer (2001, p. 119)

The conclusions of the hallucination argument differently expressed, more relevantly to our concerns, are that the alternative to phenomenalism and indirect realism is wrong. That alternative is naïve or direct realism.

Honderich (2014, p. 359)

We should note that the object of a perception, on our analysis of perceptual acquaintance and acquaintance sense, is an ordinary physical or natural object and not an unusual 'phenomenal' object or a 'sense-datum.' Thus our analysis is committed to 'direct' or 'naïve' realism, if that view is, as Romane Clark has characterized it, simply the thesis that the objects of perception are everyday physical objects.

Smith and McIntyre (1984, pp. 365–366)

In that sense, Plato's suggestion that under appropriate conditions mind-independent reality can be directly grasped is analogous to the more familiar direct, or naïve realism.

Rockmore (2011, p. 9)

According to the phenomenalist, perception consists in having the sense-data: there is no mediation, because there are no 'external,' mind-independent things. The other standard approach to perception is direct (or naïve) realism.

McCullough (1994, p. 87)

Metaphysical Realism (…) has an epistemological component, which is divided into two main categories: direct (or naïve) realism and representative (or causal) realism.

Stroll (2000, p. 96)

APPENDIX B

Some additional representative examples of the underspecification of Naïve Realism include the following.

According to Logue (2012, p. 173), Naïve Realism "is a theory about *veridical* experience—the sort of experience in which a subject perceives things, and they appear to the subject to have certain properties because the subject *perceives* those properties… What Naïve Realism says about veridical perceptual experience is that it *fundamentally consists in the subject perceiving things in her environment and some of their properties.*" (The italicization here is hers.)

According to Nudds (2009, p. 355), "Naïve Realism is the view that veridical perceptual experiences have a phenomenal character that consists of relations to mind-independent objects and features."

Characterizations of Naïve Realism as an account of veridical perceptual experience such as those given, respectively, by Logue and Nudds, characterizations typically found in the literature, lump under "veridical" perceptual experience both objectual and qualitative veridicality. Doing so betrays a tendency, widespread in the literature, to lump together under "Naïve Realism" various Naïve Realisms worth explicitly distinguishing.

REFERENCES

Alston, W.P., 1999. Back to the theory of appearing. Philos. Perspect. 13, 181–203.
Beck, L.W., 1966. 18th Century Philosophy. The Free Press, New York.
Broad, C.D., 1914. Perception, Physics, and Reality. Cambridge University Press, Cambridge.
Bunge, M., 1977. Treatise on Basic Philosophy, vol. 3. Reidel, Dordrecht.
Campbell, J., 2002. Reference and Consciousness. Oxford University Press, Oxford.
Fish, W., 2009. Perception, Hallucination, and Illusion. Oxford University Press, Oxford.
Fish, W., 2010. Philosophy of Perception: A Contemporary Introduction. Routledge, New York, NY.
Honderich, T., 2014. Actual Consciousness. Oxford University Press, Oxford.
Huemer, M., 2001. Skepticism and the Veil of Perception. Rowman & Littlefield, Lanham, MD.
Le Morvan, P., 2008. Sensory experience and intentionalism. Philos. Compass 3, 1–18.
Logue, H., 2012. What should the naïve realist say about total hallucinations? Philos. Perspect. 26, 173–199.
Martin, M.G.F., 2004. The limits of self-awareness. Philos. Stud. 120, 37–89.
McCullough, G., 1994. Using Sartre. Routledge, New York.

Nudds, M., 2009. Recent work in perception: naïve realism and its opponents. Analysis 69 (2), 334–346.

Paulsen, F., Thilly, F., 1895. Introduction to Philosophy. Henry Holt and Company, New York.

Price, H.H., 1932. Perception. Methuen, London.

Pronin, E., Gilovich, T., Ross, L., 2004. Objectivity in the eye of the beholder: divergent perceptions of bias in self versus others. Psychol. Rev. 111 (3), 781–799.

Rockmore, T., 2011. Kant and Phenomenology. University of Chicago Press, Chicago.

Satel, S., Lilienfeld, S., 2013. Brainwashed: The Seductive Appeal of Mindless Neuroscience. Basic Books, New York.

Smith, D.W., McIntyre, R., 1984. Husserl and Intentionality. Reidel, Dordrecht.

Stroll, A., 2000. Twentieth-Century Analytic Philosophy. Columbia University Press, New York.

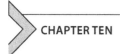

CHAPTER TEN

A Dilemma for Epistemological Disjunctivism

Eva Schmidt
Philosophy Department, University of Zürich (UZH), Zürich, Switzerland

1. INTRODUCTION

In this chapter, I argue that epistemological disjunctivism, a view defended by Pritchard (2012) or McDowell (1982/2009), faces a dilemma. The epistemological disjunctivist, if she does not want to accept the "highest common factor view" (McDowell, 1982/2009, p. 80)—to which her position is supposed to be a genuine alternative—has to endorse a metaphysical brand of disjunctivism as well. This is so because her claim that veridical perception provides the perceiver with reflectively accessible epistemic reasons that are superior to those provided by hallucination is plausible only if it is underwritten by the naïve realist claim that perception is partly constituted by the perceived fact. As I argue, this claim leads inexorably to metaphysical disjunctivism. So, epistemological disjunctivism cannot be advertised as a view that shares some of the advantages of metaphysical disjunctivism but is less extreme and therefore more widely acceptable than the latter view.

In the following, I will first introduce the relevant views of perceptual experience and some important concepts. Next, I will set up the dilemma and defend each of its horns. I will close by discussing and rejecting one route of escape for the epistemological disjunctivist.

Let me start with some terminology. I use "perception" and "perceive" exclusively to refer to cases of veridical perception, where all goes well. My term for the mental state that is allegedly present in perception, hallucination, and illusion is "perceptual experience." The "good case" is the case in which the subject perceives; the "bad case" is the case in which the subject undergoes a hallucination. Illusion will not play a role in my discussion. In the literature, it is sometimes classified with perception as a kind of good case and sometimes with hallucination as a kind of bad case, an issue I will not take a stand on here.

Direct versus Indirect Realism
ISBN 978-0-12-812141-2
https://doi.org/10.1016/B978-0-12-812141-2.00010-6
141

Epistemological disjunctivism is a reaction to the traditionalist highest common factor view, which starts from the following plausible claim: For each good case of perception, it is possible that there is a bad case of hallucination, which is introspectively indistinguishable for the subject. The highest common factor view concludes from this that the subjectively accessible epistemic reasons that perception provides for empirical belief can be no better than those provided by an indistinguishable hallucination. This move can be understood as a variation on the argument from hallucination. In McDowell's words,

> since there can be deceptive cases experientially indistinguishable from non-deceptive cases, one's experiential intake – what one embraces within the scope of one's consciousness – must be the same in both kinds of case. In a deceptive case, one's experiential intake must ex hypothesi fall short of the fact itself, in the sense of being consistent with there being no such fact. So that must be true, according to the argument, in a non-deceptive case too.
>
> **McDowell (1982/2009, p. 80)**

For instance, when Louis hallucinates that there is a red box in front of him, his reason to believe that there is a red box in front of him is on a par with his reason for the same belief when he *sees* that there is a red box in front of him. In both cases, all Louis can acquire as a basis for his belief is an appearance, the visual content that there is a red box in front of him. That he has this visual appearance does not *entail* or *guarantee* that there is a red box in front of him. So even when he really is facing a red box, seeing it, his perceptual reason for his belief that there is a red box in front of him does not guarantee its truth, and it enjoys justification of the same strength as the same belief in the bad case of hallucination. (Note that I present the contents of perceptual experience in propositional form and perception as concerned with facts. My arguments can without difficulty be reformulated for views that conceive of perception as nonpropositional or nonfactual, for instance, as directed at objects. I use the propositional formulation of the contents of perceptual experience here merely for ease of exposition.)

Because of its weak conception of reasons, the highest common factor view is vulnerable to skepticism, or so McDowell (1994, p. 112/113) and Pritchard (2012, p. 118) argue. McDowell's line of thought, stated very briefly and crudely, is that to endorse the highest common factor view is to endorse fallibilism—even if the world cooperates and things are as they appear, we do not have perceptual reasons for our most fundamental beliefs about the world that are incompatible with the possibility of error. This feature of fallibilism allows skeptics to argue that our perceptual reasons do not give support to the belief that things are largely as they strike us to be, over the hypothesis that we are, say, brains in vats or the victims of an evil demon. Proponents of the common factor view, then, are unable to block the skeptical argument outright.

The highest common factor view is naturally construed not only just as a view about perceptual reasons but also as involving a claim about the nature of experience, viz. that perception and hallucination are mental states of the same (fundamental) kind. In either case, people undergo *perceptual experiences* with a certain phenomenal character (and plausibly, content). It is an additional matter whether things really are the way that experience presents them to be to the subject, i.e., whether the experience is a perception or a hallucination. This way of putting the highest common factor view fits with representationalism, which, I take it, is the most commonly held variety of the view these days. Note, however, that sense-datum theory or qualia theory are also versions of the highest common factor view.

Epistemological disjunctivists reject the assumption of the highest common factor view that the subject's epistemic reasons in the good case and in the bad case are on a par. In the good case, perception provides the subject with what I call *excellent* epistemic reasons—reasons *entailing* the truth of corresponding beliefs about the world. For instance, Louis's *seeing* that there is a red box entails that there is a red box in front of him; his belief that there is a red box in front of him is guaranteed to be true, given what he sees. In seeing, Louis takes up the fact that there is a red box in front of him; his epistemic reason is given from his subjective perspective, it is reflectively accessible to him. Epistemological disjunctivism allows for a strong antiskeptical stance. If perceivers have an immediate conscious grasp on the facts, if perception provides them with accessible reasons that guarantee the truth of basic empirical beliefs, then there is no cause to worry about skeptical possibilities—they are already excluded.

The phrase "reflectively accessible" is from Pritchard (2012, p. 13). The same idea is endorsed by Rödl (2010) and by McDowell (2011, 2013). McDowell (2013, p. 148/49) says that "the warrant-constituting status of the experience must be part of the content of an at least implicit self-consciousness." When someone has perceptual knowledge, she "must be in a position to know the warrant by virtue of which her state counts as knowledge" (McDowell, 2013, p. 148). When the subject knows that *p* by perceiving that *p*, she is in a position to know that this is so. This is an internalist notion, on which knowledge presupposes that the excellent reasons supporting her belief are accessible to the subject. It comes down to the claim that perception is a *luminous* mental state, which is to say that if the subject perceives that *p* (where this is her excellent reason supporting her belief), then she is in a position to know that she perceives that *p* (cf. Williamson, 2000; Haddock, 2013). Moreover, knowledge by perception is luminous: If the subject knows that *p* by perception, then she is in a position to know that she knows that *p* by perception.

At the same time, it is arguably possible to endorse epistemological disjunctivism while rejecting a disjunctivist view about the *nature of experience* (taken by Hinton, 1967/2009; Martin, 2004; Fish, 2009; Logue, 2012; among others). Crucially, according to *metaphysical* disjunctivist views, there is no common mental state type—perceptual experience—of which both perception and hallucination are instances. Metaphysical disjunctivism is motivated by an endorsement of *naïve realism*, the view that perception is (partly) constituted by the fact that the subject is confronted with or, similarly, that perception is a relation between the perceiver and the perceived fact. (This is relationalism, a variant of naïve realism.) It is by its very nature a confrontation with worldly facts, a kind of mental state that it is impossible to undergo in the absence of the perceived fact. Further, according to naïve realism, the subjective character of perception is partly supplied by the qualities of the things themselves that are perceived.[1]

The metaphysical disjunctivist's claims about perception are obviously not true of hallucination. *It* is not a relation to a fact, which provides for the hallucinatory phenomenal character. Whatever we can say to characterize hallucination, the lesson that the naïve realist *cum* metaphysical disjunctivist takes from this is that we will not be able to find any substantial commonalities between hallucination and perception, which would then warrant classifying both types of mental state as belonging to the mental state type *perceptual experience*. This is not to deny that there may be uninteresting features shared by these two kinds of mental state, for instance, that they are both indistinguishable from perception (Martin, 2004) or that they are mental states. Another feature they may have in common is that they play similar causal roles (e.g., that they lead to similar beliefs or behavior).

---

[1] As a side note, be aware that naïve realism is not the same as direct realism, but is rather one specific version of it. Direct realism subsumes other views as well, for instance representationalism, the view that perceptual experience is essentially a representation of the subject's environment. According to direct realism, we immediately perceive things in our environment. This contrasts with *indirect* realism, the view that our perception of worldly objects is mediated by sense-data or the like, which are (typically conceived as) mental entities that are immediately present to us in perceptual experience.

There are several ways of spelling out disjunctivist views of this metaphysical variety, and it is not easy to determine which of them is the best. (For my project in this chapter, this contributes to the following tension: On the one hand, one ought not to saddle the metaphysical disjunctivist with an implausibly ambitious view. But on the other hand, I should not make things too easy for myself by weakening metaphysical disjunctivism so much that epistemological disjunctivism is burdened with it without further ado. I will address this issue at the end of the chapter.) Byrne and Logue (2008) insist that the only genuine metaphysical disjunctivism holds that there is *no* common mental element had by perception and hallucination. Another standard formulation of disjunctivism about the nature of experience is Martin's (2004), who holds (merely) that perception and hallucination do not share the same *fundamental* kind. In deciding on a particular formulation there are two things to keep in mind. First, metaphysical disjunctivism's *raison d'être* is to uphold naïve realism or a relational view about perception. Perception is a relation to a fact, which is what its phenomenal character is (partly) due to. Second, metaphysical disjunctivism is interested in rejecting the traditional view that there is a common mental state, called "perceptual experience," shared by perception and hallucination. Since its phenomenal character is an essential feature of a perceptual experience, this gives us a commitment to the claim that there is no phenomenal character in common between perception and hallucination. (For otherwise there would certainly be a common state, deserving of the title "perceptual experience.")

As a result of these considerations, the claim I take here to be definitive of metaphysical disjunctivism is that *there is no true shared characterization of perception and hallucination that captures something essential about and specific to both, especially none in terms of their phenomenal character.* My shorthand for this will be: There are no substantial commonalities between perception and hallucination.

2. THE DILEMMA FOR EPISTEMOLOGICAL DISJUNCTIVISM

There is general consent that the epistemological disjunctivist is not committed to metaphysical disjunctivism (see Byrne and Logue, 2008; Soteriou, 2014; McDowell, 2008; Haddock and Macpherson, 2008; Snowdon, 2005. For dissenting voices, see Littlejohn, 2016; Cunningham, 2016). Rather, she can allow that there *are* substantial commonalities between perception and hallucination, for instance, that they are mental states of the same fundamental kind or that they have an interesting mental element in common. For example, McDowell (2008, p. 382) holds that a "difference in epistemic significance is of course consistent with all sorts of commonalities between the disjuncts [such as that] it appears to one that, say, there is a red cube in front of one." Pritchard (2012, p. 24) claims that epistemological disjunctivism "does not entail that there is no common metaphysical essence to the experiences of the agent [in perception and hallucination.]" The following two conditions have to be met by epistemological disjunctivism *sans* metaphysical disjunctivism:

> (ExR) In the good case, but not in the indistinguishable bad case, the subject possesses a reflectively accessible excellent reason to believe that p in virtue of perceiving that p.

This epistemic difference is supposedly compatible with the claim that

> (SubC) Perception and hallucination have substantial commonalities.

I disagree. I maintain that proponents of epistemological disjunctivism are forced to endorse metaphysical disjunctivism as well. I will next argue for my claim by presenting a dilemma for the epistemological disjunctivist. The dilemma is that she can meet condition (ExR) only at the price of burdening herself with metaphysical disjunctivism (not meeting condition (SubC)) and can meet condition (SubC) only at the price of collapsing into the highest common factor view (not meeting condition (ExR)). Since her view is supposed to provide a genuine alternative to the highest common factor view, her only option, then, is to endorse metaphysical disjunctivism. The cost of this move is that many find metaphysical disjunctivism completely untenable—in Searle's (2015, p. 180) harsh words, "the [metaphysical] Disjunctivist conception of perception is not so much false as incoherent." I will conclude the paper by presenting (and rebutting) the most promising defense of the epistemological disjunctivist against my attack.

2.1 Excellent Reasons Preclude Substantial Commonalities

Condition (ExR) requires there to be something that is an excellent reason to believe that *p*, which is missing in the bad case and which the subject has reflective access to. More precisely, the subject's perception that *p* has to provide her with an epistemic reason to believe that *p* that guarantees that *p* is the case; moreover, the subject needs to have reflective access to this excellent reason. In the case of hallucination, the excellent reason is absent.

In thinking about what the excellent reason might be, then, in the first place, we have to find something that is present in the good case and missing in the bad case; in the second place, this something has to guarantee the truth of basic empirical belief; and finally, it has to be reflectively accessible to the subject. This excludes the perceptual experience or its content, for both are the same in the good and bad cases. Take Louis's perceptual experience that there is a red box in front of him. Granting that there is a mental state of perceptual experience common to perception and hallucination, it is going to be available to Louis in both cases as a perceptual reason. Further, it is not the kind of reason that entails that there is a red box in front of Louis—there might be *nothing* in front of him, as when he is in an empty room while hallucinating that there is a red box in front of him. (The suggestion here could be either that the subject's *perceptual experience* or that the *fact* that the subject has the perceptual experience is her epistemic reason. This distinction makes no difference for my point and will be ignored in the following.)

Nor is the common conscious content of Louis's perceptual experience a fit candidate for the epistemological disjunctivist's excellent reason. It does not meet the aforementioned requirements for excellent reasons because it is present in the good *and* the bad case. For instance, say that the content of Louis's visual experience is the proposition *that there is a red box in front of him*. This proposition is available to Louis as his epistemic reason in the bad case just as well as in the good case. Moreover, since having this kind of content is consistent with the world not being as it is represented, as in Louis's hallucination of the red box, such a reason does not guarantee that the corresponding belief is true.

Something that does fit the bill of an excellent reason in that it is unique to the good case and guarantees the truth of the relevant belief is *the fact itself* that is perceived by the subject. That there is a red box in front of Louis entails the truth of his belief that there is a red box in front of him. (Let us ignore the so-called basis problem about saying that the fact that *p* is a reason to believe that *p*. cf. Pritchard, 2012; Littlejohn, 2016.) Also, this fact is missing in the situation in which Louis hallucinates the presence of a red box in an empty room. However, this worldly fact is outside the reach of the subject's reflective access—unless we conceive of perception as the naïve realist does, viz. as partly constituted by this fact. According to a relationist formulation of naïve realism, when Louis sees that there is a red box in front of him, his seeing is a relation between him and the fact that there is a red box in front of him. Seeing essentially involves the seen fact, and it is plausible that the fact is internal (not "blankly external" McDowell, 1982/2009, p. 82) to the subject's perspective, for the perceived objects and their properties and relations contribute to the subjective character of perception, according to the naïve realist. However, this leads right to metaphysical disjunctivism, as I will argue next.

This is because epistemological disjunctivists have to accept the (independently plausible) claim that perception is transparent, i.e., that the introspectively accessible, conscious features of perception turn out not to be intrinsic qualities of the mental state itself, but rather properties of or relations between the objects presented in perception (cf. Moore, 1903/1965, p. 20; Harman, 1990, p. 39; Tye, 2000, p. 45). This commitment is needed to ascertain the directness of perception, or, in McDowell's (1982/2009, p. 84) words, the conception of perception as "openness" to the world. Think about it this way: Perception appears to present me just with the things that surround me. Now say it turns out that some of these apparent outward things or properties are indeed *intrinsic qualities* of my experience, even though as a matter of fact I cannot tell them apart from the external objects or properties also presented to me in my current experience. This casts doubt on the claim that perception provides me with reflectively accessible excellent reasons at all—how could it, given that, even as I perceive, I cannot tell what about my environment it is that I have excellent perceptual reasons to believe.

For similar reasons, it would be wrong-headed to say that the conscious features of perception go back partly to the fact presented (again the naïve realist claim) and partly to the *content* of perception, shared by hallucination. This again would deprive the perceiver of her reflective access to which features of perception provide her with excellent epistemic reasons, for she would not be able to tell which perceived features go back to the perceived fact and which to the content. Moreover, it is not clear how the presented environmental fact and the additional content are supposed to come together to constitute one unified conscious perception, in which the subject appears to be confronted with just her environment. After all, she is not aware of a perceptual content *on top of* the world she perceives.

So, given transparency and the claim that the perceived fact is the reflectively accessible excellent reason, it follows that the phenomenal character of perception is *entirely* due to the seen fact. In the case of Louis's seeing, the very redness and boxiness of the box contribute to and exhaust what it is like to see the red box. There is no room for substantial experiential commonalities between perception and hallucination, then. Endorsing the naïve realist picture of perception will move the epistemological disjunctivist right along into metaphysical disjunctivism. On the other hand, the perceived fact will not be accessible in the right way to satisfy the epistemological disjunctivist's access requirement unless it partly constitutes the subjective character of the perceiver's experience, i.e., unless we assume naïve realism.

The next candidate for the role of excellent reason is the *mental state* of perception. It is both exclusive to the good case and factive—that Louis sees that there is a red box in front of him entails that there is indeed a red box in front of him. It is also reflectively accessible to Louis that he is seeing the red box, at least if we follow McDowell's (2011, 2013) argument that just because *in the bad case*, the subject is mistaken about whether she perceives that *p*, this does not detract from the fact that *in the good case* she can and often does know that she perceives that *p*.

However, this line of thought is available to the epistemological disjunctivist only if she conceives of perception as a genuine, nonhybrid mental state (cf. Pritchard, 2012, p. 38). On a hybrid or composite conception of perception, perceiving is having a perceptual experience as of *p* plus *p*'s being the case *plus* *p*'s having caused the perceptual experience in the right way. Unsurprisingly, this conjunctive state of affairs is factive—after all, the fact that *p* is added on to the experience. However, taking the subject's perspective, all that is internal or reflectively accessible is the visual experience itself, i.e., a mental state that is common to hallucination and perception. The fact that *p* is extra to the perceptual experience that *p*, on this conception, and so is also extra to what the subject can access or be aware of by reflection alone. On the other hand, if perception is construed as a noncomposite state, as essentially a relation to the perceived fact, we are right back with naïve realism and, by the argument just given (when discussing the perceived fact as excellent reason), with metaphysical disjunctivism: Given that the perceived fact exhausts what is conscious about perception, it is hard to see how there could be any more than superficial commonalities between it and hallucination.

This gets me to the final candidate for the role of an excellent reason, the content of perception, which some take to be a kind of content that is necessarily absent from hallucination or, respectively, to involve content elements that are necessarily lacking in hallucination. The paradigmatic example of this is Tye's (2009, p 80) "Singular (When Filled)" content, which is a singular content involving particular objects in the case of perception, but something like a Russellian proposition that contains slots instead of particular objects in hallucination.[2] So, Louis sees that *that* red box is in front of him, but he only hallucinates that __ is in front of him. (His hallucination has a content, but it is not a singular content involving the particular red box.) The epistemological disjunctivist could then insist that perception has a content that entails the truth of basic empirical belief, which hallucination lacks. She could point out that the singular Russellian proposition *that that red box is in front of Louis* really just is the fact that the particular red box is in front of Louis. This fact, which is the content of Louis's seeing, entails that there is a red box in front of him. As the content of his perception, it is unproblematically reflectively accessible to him. Nonetheless, it could be claimed, perception and hallucination have substantial commonalities in that their contents partly overlap and in that they are both relations to (something like) a Russellian proposition.

I am not convinced. If we grant that, in perception, subjects are confronted with particular facts, we have already bought into the naïve realist picture of perception on which perception is a relation between perceiver and perceived fact. On the other hand, as Tye (2009, p. 81) says, in hallucination, the subject hallucinates "something," but whatever this strange gappy something may be, I do not see that it could be of the same kind as a tangible, concrete fact that is presented in perception. There is then a difference between the contents of perception and the contents of hallucination that is as stark as ever. While seeing relates Louis to a fact, hallucinating is just a relation to an elusive something; plausibly, there is no substantial commonality between these two kinds of mental states.

There is a view in the neighborhood of Tye's that is defended, e.g., by Sosa (2011), Johnston (2004/2009), and Schmidt (2015), according to which the content or object shared by perception and hallucination consists in uninstantiated qualities (e.g., the qualities of being red, cubical, in a certain location, etc.). The content (or object) that is particular to perception, by contrast, consists in these qualities *also being instantiated*. Johnston (2004/2009, p. 226) holds that, in the good case, you are "visually aware of

---

[2] To elucidate, Russellian propositions, by contrast with Fregean propositions, are structured complexes that involve the worldly objects thought about themselves. For instance, the Russellian proposition *that there is that red box*, as asserted by Louis, has the red box in front of him itself as a constituent. The notion goes back to Bertrand Russell, who contends, in correspondence with Frege: "I believe that in spite of all its snowfields Mont Blanc itself is a component part of what is actually asserted in the proposition 'Mont Blanc is more than 4000 metres high'. We do not assert the thought, for this is a private psychological matter: we assert the object of the thought, and this is, to my mind, a certain complex (an objective proposition, one might say) in which Mont Blanc is itself a component part" (Frege, 1980, p. 169). Fregean propositions are structured complexes of Fregean senses or modes of presentation of worldly entities.

a host of spatio-temporal particulars instantiating parts of such a... complex of sensible qualities and relations." Here, again, the epistemological disjunctivist might hope that the represented qualities are what perception and hallucination have in common, whereas the instantiation of these qualities, represented only by perception, can be identified as the accessible excellent reason that is unique to the good case. Why is this reason an excellent reason? The instantiation of the perceived qualities plausibly gives us a worldly fact. If this fact is included in perception, it is guaranteed that what is believed is the case.

While I myself am very sympathetic to an account of perceptual content along these lines, I do not think that we can here find an accessible excellent reason that is available to the subject only in the good case. It is true that the correctness of perception is provided by the instantiation of the represented qualities, and that this account avoids commitment to a problematic veil of perception. Still, in what sense does it allow for the subject to have reflective access to the fact itself, which consists in the relevant particulars instantiating the qualities represented by perceptual experience? Plausibly, the reflectively accessible content of perception and hallucination both consists in the complex of sensible qualities; this is what makes up the subjective character of perceptual experience *in its entirety*. Whether these qualities are also instantiated goes beyond what it is like for the subject, and thus also beyond her reflective grasp. (Perceptual experience is transparent—but how could it be transparent to both the complex of sensible qualities, which is an abstract object, and to the concrete fact that is an instantiation of these qualities? When I focus on what I am seeing right now, for instance, I do not find myself focusing on a complex abstract object and, on top of that, on a worldly fact.) I conclude that this conception of perceptual content is not available to the epistemological disjunctivist. Overall, the prospects of this strategy—identifying the excellent reasons provided by perception with the special content of perception—are dim.

A somewhat different way to develop this kind of proposal might be to identify perceptual contents with object-dependent Fregean propositions. An object-dependent or *de re* Fregean sense (like *that box*) is a mode of presentation of a particular object, which depends, for its existence, on the existence of the object it picks out (the particular box) (cf. Evans, 1982; McDowell, 1984, 1998.). A Fregean proposition that involves an object-dependent Fregean sense (like the proposition *that that box is red*) is itself object-dependent. A necessary condition on the existence of such a proposition is that the particular object involved in the fact, which is picked out by the proposition, exists. But note that the mere existence of an object-dependent proposition does not guarantee that it is true; for instance, the proposition *that that box is green* exists even if that box is red. So, that the subject's perception has an object-dependent proposition as its content is not by itself sufficient to guarantee the truth of the corresponding belief. What would guarantee its truth is the truth of the perceptual content. However, for the truth of the object-dependent proposition to be a part of the reflectively accessible perceptual reason, it seems that the *fact* that makes the proposition true would have to be reflectively accessible to the subject. And as I have argued, this gets us right back to metaphysical disjunctivism.

From my discussion of the perceived fact, the mental state of perception and the content of perception as the subject's excellent reasons, we can extract a general problem of the attempt to combine (ExR), the thesis that there are reflectively accessible, excellent reasons that are unique to perception, with (SubC), the claim that it has substantial commonalities with hallucination: According to (ExR), perception involves a reason that is both accessible to the subject and unique to the good case. What is reflectively accessible about a perception is how it presents the world to the perceiver. Given the epistemological disjunctivist's commitment to transparency, this just is the phenomenal character of the experience. So the reason that is unique to the good case plausibly exhausts what is conscious to the subject about her perception. There is then no room for significant commonalities between perception and hallucination with respect to what it is like to undergo them: What is conscious about perception is unique to the good case; whatever it may be that supplies the subjective character of hallucination, it must be of a completely different nature.[3]

It is true that when the subject undergoes an introspectively indistinguishable hallucination, the world *appears* to be the same to her as in the corresponding perception. But given that it simply cannot involve the something that is unique to perception, which, according to my argument, exhausts the conscious character of that mental state, it has to be of a completely different kind. The point that the world *appears* to be the same in the good and the bad cases comes to nothing more than what a defender of metaphysical disjunctivism like Martin is claiming

---

[3] As this indicates, my argument is not committed to conceiving of perception as propositional. What I need is only that there is something (propositional or not) that is the epistemic reason, which is excellent, unique to the good case, and reflectively accessible. This gives us naïve realism, and adding the transparency of experience, we arrive at metaphysical disjunctivism.

anyway—viz., that she cannot introspectively distinguish these two situations. It does not amount to the claim that perception and hallucination have any substantial commonalities. (This deals with Byrne and Logue's (2008) claim that the mental state of *looking* a certain way is a substantial commonality between perception and hallucination, and also with McDowell's idea that there are two kinds of appearances, viz. mere appearances and perceptually manifest facts, which share the common kind of being appearances.)

Overall, no matter how we approach the issue, via the fact presented, the mental state of perception, or its special content, condition (ExR) is met only if perception is partly constituted by the perceived fact (i.e., if naïve realism is true). Together with transparency, this has the consequence that perception and hallucination do not have any substantial experiential commonalities, and that (SubC) is not met.

2.2 Substantial Commonalities Preclude Excellent Reasons

But what if we approach the issue from the opposite direction? Maybe we can insist on the truth of (SubC), that is, claim that there are significant mental commonalities between perception and hallucination, and at the same time eke out some room for reflectively accessible excellent reasons that are unique to perception (that is, the truth of (ExR)). Let me now show that this strategy is also unsuccessful.

Possible candidates for what perception and hallucination may have in common are the *mental state* of perceptual experience and their shared representational *content*. To start with the first possibility, can we insist that there is a shared mental state of perceptual experience, but then also allow for the truth of (ExR)? As I have argued above, if we want to take seriously the idea that perception and hallucination involve the very same kind of mental state, we cannot maintain that this state is a relation between the perceiver and the perceived fact. Still, it might be that two mental states of the same kind have contents of different kinds. But if the content that p of a perception is to be the excellent good case reason, it has to guarantee the truth of the belief that p. Also, this has to be reflectively accessible to the perceiver. Again, I do not see how this could be the case unless the content of perception is identified with the perceived fact. And this claim turns perception into a relation to the perceived fact, so that we lose any substantial commonalities between the mental states of perception and of hallucination.

What then about the second possibility, that the commonality between perception and hallucination consists in their shared content? McDowell (2013, p. 147) suggests:

An experience that is a seeing can be like an experience that merely appears to put its subject in touch with a corresponding environmental reality in respect of what content it has. But a seeing is unlike a mere appearing in how it has its content. Seeings have their content in a way that is characteristic of seeings; they make environmental realities present to the subject.

What can be extracted from this quote is that indistinguishable perception and hallucination have the same content, on McDowell's view. On p. 154, he suggests that both "have their content determined by their being, among other things, acts of a capacity to have [the relevant worldly features perceptually] present to one...." But this leaves it open that the content is present in different ways. In perception, it is presented in such a way that it is guaranteed, from the subject's perspective, that what is perceived is the case—an environmental reality is genuinely made present to the perceiver. In hallucination, by contrast, the subject is merely *apparently* put in touch with a worldly fact. So there is an excellent reason uniquely available in the good case, thanks to the relation to the facts that perception manages to establish to the world. Still, the subject exercises the same capacity to have her environment perceptually present in both cases; it is just that she exercises this capacity successfully in the good case and unsuccessfully in the bad case. Assuming that the capacity exercised fixes the content, both the good case and the bad case involve the same kind of content. This suffices to give us the truth of (SubC) together with the truth of (ExR).

Here is my objection: Assume that the same kind of content really is involved in perception and hallucination that *p*. Additionally, grant that the former, but not the latter, is the success case of having the content. The problem for the claim that this gives us an excellent, reflectively accessible reason that is unique to the good case is that it is not clear how the fact that she is in the success case can be *reflectively accessible* to the perceiver, given the assumption. For it to be so, it would seem that the worldly fact that perception reaches out to and puts the subject in touch with has to be accessible to her. This is not possible under the assumption that the mental states of perception and hallucination are both just instances of a mental state—an exercise of a capacity to have the environment perceptually present to one—*with the very same content*. Rather, it would require perception to have the perceived fact itself as its content, which is unique to the good case, instead of having the same content as hallucination. To back this up, note that it cannot be the case that perception is a relation to the fact that p, such that the fact is *not* the content of the perception, but still it is reflectively accessible to the perceiver that it is such a relation. For assume that seeing that there is a red box and hallucinating that there is a red box is genuinely subjectively the same for Louis with respect to what is represented to him. Then there simply is no room for an additional, reflectively accessible feature unique to seeing that might provide his access to the fact that he is in the success case. Moreover, as before, it cannot be right that, in perception, both the fact and the shared content are transparently present to the perceiver as how the world strikes her. For she is not aware of two distinct things that are given in perception, the fact and the content, but only of one. All this goes to show that, given the truth of (SubC) as spelled out on the current proposal, there is no room for excellent reasons that are reflectively accessible to the perceiver in the good case (ExR).

Importantly, my point is not that epistemological disjunctivism requires an *infallible* capacity to know by perception (which McDowell, 2011; Rödl, 2010, for instance, rightly reject). It is, merely, that there is no room for the subject to be reflectively aware of her perceptual relation to her environment, given that the subjective character of both perception and hallucination is exhausted by their shared content.

Let me conclude that the epistemological disjunctivist cannot endorse (SubC) without losing hold of (ExR), that is, without collapsing into the highest common factor view. No matter where we posit substantial commonalities between perception and hallucination—in the mental state of perceptual experience or in its content—we find that it precludes the subject from having reflectively accessible excellent epistemic reasons that are unique to the good case.

3. AN ESCAPE ROUTE?

So far, I have tried my hardest to settle the epistemological disjunctivist with metaphysical disjunctivism. However, I think that there is another line that the epistemological disjunctivist might push, which is not so obviously doomed to fail: Maybe there is a way to maintain, first, that the mental states of perception and of hallucination share substantial commonalities, and second that perceiving that p guarantees the truth of a belief that p in a way that is reflectively accessible to the perceiver. I am thinking here of a conception of perceptual experience and perception modeled on Williamson's (2000) account of believing and knowing, according to which, in a sense, "[k]nowing is… the best kind of believing. Mere believing is a kind of botched knowing." (Williamson, 2000, p. 47) (Also note the similarities with the just discussed McDowell, 2013.) Transferring this picture to perception, we have to take perception, a *factive* mental state, as our conceptual starting point. This is the optimal variety of perceptual experience, in which we are in touch with our surroundings. But there are other varieties of perceptual experience, in which things are going suboptimally, i.e., types of mere perceptual experience, among them hallucination. Hallucination, then, is a kind of "botched" perception.

It seems that this picture of perception gets the epistemological disjunctivist what she needs: Perception is factive, so a perception that *p* guarantees that a belief that *p* based on it is true. The epistemological disjunctivist might even be able to insist that perception is not partly constituted by the perceived fact (at least not in any threatening sense). It might be argued that the factivity of perception comes down to the fact that "perception" is a success noun, which we only employ in descriptions of situations in which the subject does manage to get in touch with the world. There is simply no need to draw conclusions about the metaphysics of the mental state of perception! Further, it is unproblematic to allow that perception and hallucination are instances of the same mental kind on this picture. They are both varieties of perception, where the one just *is* perception, and the other is perception gone awry. The last ingredient to this account is the plausible claim that the perceiver's excellent reason, perception, *is* reflectively accessible to the perceiver, for it is a conscious, occurrent mental state. It seems undeniable that the perceiver's own conscious, occurrent mental states are not blankly external to her perspective. The epistemological disjunctivist can here repeat the point that the subject's inability to tell in the bad case that she is merely hallucinating should not be seen to detract from the fact that she knows in the good case that she is perceiving. So we get the mental state of perception that satisfies both (ExR) and (SubC): Perception can be identified as the reflectively accessible, excellent reason that is unique to the good case but is instantiated in the bad case in a suboptimal way.

Admittedly, this framework appears much more amenable to the epistemological disjunctivist's interests. Leaving to one side the concern (to my mind not fully dispelled) that the subject will not be able to reflectively access the fact that she is perceiving on this picture,[4] here is a further

---

[4] Williamson (2000, pp. 11–13), for one, rejects the claim that knowledge is luminous in this way. So for him, the subject does not meet the internalist reflective access requirement. Cf. Pritchard (2011).

problem that blocks the epistemological disjunctivist's escape route: In this framework, the only thing allowed to play the role of excellent reason, the only thing that can ever give rise to the subject's excellent epistemic justification, which is able to block the skeptical argument outright, is her own mental state of perception. For instance, the exclusive source of Louis's excellent justification for his belief that there is a red box in front of him is his *seeing* that there is a red box in front of him.

But this is implausible. What the epistemological disjunctivist (rightly) wants is that, in the good case, the world itself contributes to the excellent justification of our beliefs about the world. What makes the justification of Louis's belief unshakable is *the worldly fact* that there is a red box in front of him. If challenged, one reason that Louis might plausible provide for thinking that there is a red box in front of him is just that there *is* a red box in front of him. The framework currently under discussion cannot do justice to this role of *worldly facts* rather than (facts about) mental states. Epistemological disjunctivism thereby loses some of its antiskeptical appeal: On the current approach, it's not the world itself that contributes to my excellent epistemic standing, but only my own mental states.

Here is another way to illustrate the problem: When Louis sees that the child is drowning, he can answer both the question, "what is your reason to believe the child is drowning?" and the question "what is your reason to jump in the water?" by saying, "just look, the child is drowning." Thereby, he makes reference not to the fact that he *sees* that the child is drowning, but to the fact, which perception makes available to him, that the child is drowning. (Plausibly, he tries to direct his interlocutor's attention to this fact by replying in this way.) The fact justifies both his belief that the child is drowning and his action of jumping in. What counts in favor of Louis's jumping in the water to save the child is not his mental state, but the fact that the child is drowning; this very fact also counts in favor of his believing that the child is drowning. Moreover, what motivates Louis to jump in the water is that the child is drowning, not his perception of her drowning; and similarly, we should allow that what moves him to believe that the child is drowning is that she is drowning, as a matter of fact (cf. Dancy, 2000; Hornsby, 2008). To be clear, my point concerning reasons to believe is not that it is false that the mental state of perception (or the fact that the subject perceives) is an excellent reason to have corresponding beliefs. It is that the very fact that is perceived may also be an excellent reason to believe something, which the epistemological disjunctivist cannot allow, on the current proposal.

So, the escape route is blocked because it excludes one class of excellent epistemic reasons—worldly facts—that, plausibly, the epistemological disjunctivist should allow. So in the end, appealing to a factive state of perception while rejecting naïve realism cannot save epistemological disjunctivism sans metaphysical disjunctivism.

For a final comeback, the epistemological disjunctivist might stick with the idea that the required substantial commonality consists in the shared mental state—that both perception and hallucination are a kind of perception, or in McDowell's terms, an exercise of the same capacity. She could then insist that only the success case of perception makes the perceived fact reflectively available, and that this perceived fact is the excellent reason. Even if it exhausts the subjective character of perception, so that there are no phenomenal commonalities between perception and hallucination, this leaves the possibility that they have substantial commonalities, which are not conscious and to which the subject has *no* reflective access. According to this last comeback, the relevant commonality is that perception and hallucination are both (optimal or botched, as the case may be) varieties of perception or exercises of a capacity to know by perceiving. All the epistemological disjunctivist needs to do to save her view is to concede that this commonality is not reflectively available to the subject.

This may well be the most promising epistemological disjunctivist proposal. Does this commit the proponents of this view to metaphysical disjunctivism? Recall the motivations for metaphysical disjunctivism I elucidated in Section 1. First off, metaphysical disjunctivists defend the idea that perception and hallucination share no phenomenal character. This is to make sure the perceived fact supplies the phenomenal character of perception. The epistemological disjunctivist proposal under consideration concedes this. To the extent that this is all that metaphysical disjunctivism wants to achieve, the proposal *is* a version of metaphysical disjunctivism (cf. Cunningham, 2016, p. 113). The same goes for Martin's (2004) view that perception and hallucination are mental states of different fundamental kinds. Perception is most fundamentally a relation to a fact. This is compatible with its also being, such as hallucination, an exercise of a capacity to know by perceiving, as long this is not as fundamental.

But secondly, metaphysical disjunctivism aims to reject the existence of a mental state of perceptual experience and so can be understood as denying that there are *any* substantial commonalities between perception and hallucination whatsoever (not limited to ones that are conscious or reflectively accessible). To the extent that this is also part of the metaphysical disjunctivist project, the current proposal disagrees: It insists that there is a true shared characterization of perception and hallucination that captures something essential about and specific to both, viz. their characterization as (optimal or botched) instances of perception, or as exercises of a capacity to know by perception. The epistemological disjunctivist may contend that this goes to show that she endorses the existence of a genuine mental state of perceptual experience and thus stops short of metaphysical disjunctivism.

Let me give a diagnostic comment before turning to problems of this comeback. Should we construe metaphysical disjunctivism in such a strong way that it denies the existence even of reflectively inaccessible substantial commonalities that do not relate to the phenomenal character of perception and hallucination? My uneasy position here is that I should not make my case against epistemological disjunctivism too easy, but also should not settle the metaphysical disjunctivist with a view that is implausibly demanding. I am not sure how to resolve this tension. Instead, let me record that, minimally, my argument shows that epistemological disjunctivism is committed to *some* varieties of metaphysical disjunctivism.

Even beyond this, the proposal comes at a cost. For one, the epistemological disjunctivist has to tell the following, highly implausible story: Indistinguishable perceptions and hallucinations appear to have the same phenomenal character to the subject. But this is deceiving, according to the proposal—they do not. For the phenomenal character of perception goes back to the fact perceived, and no such thing is true of hallucination. Still, as it happens, perception and hallucination are mental states of the same type—they are both instances of the mental state of perception or, respectively, both exercises of a capacity to know by perception. But the subject is introspectively completely in the dark about *this* commonality.

For another, the claim that the proposed commonalities are sufficient for establishing that perception and hallucination fall under the mental state type *perceptual experience* is untenable. Here is why: Its phenomenal character is essential for a particular type of perceptual experience. Any perceptual experience of this type must therefore have this same phenomenal character. But according to the epistemological disjunctivist comeback, perception and hallucination, although of the same kind, share no phenomenal character. So whatever mental kind they fall under, it cannot be the kind *perceptual experience.* In light of this, I don't see what should stop metaphysical disjunctivists from allowing the commonality, seeing as it does not conflict with their motivation of getting rid of the mental state of perceptual experience.

All in all, then, even this last attempt to evade the dilemma is highly problematic. I conclude that those who endorse epistemological disjunctivism also have to accept some versions of metaphysical disjunctivism. If my last line of thought is correct, they even have to accept all plausible versions of metaphysical disjunctivism.

4. UPSHOT

In this paper, I have argued that epistemological disjunctivism cannot be upheld without incurring a commitment to metaphysical disjunctivism as well. The dilemma for the epistemological disjunctivist is that to reject metaphysical disjunctivism is to endorse (SubC), the claim that there are substantial commonalities between perception and hallucination. But endorsing (SubC) comes down to endorsing the highest common factor view—it leaves no room for reflectively accessible excellent reasons that are unique to the good case. On the other hand, I have argued, the claim that distinguishes epistemological disjunctivism from the highest common factor view, (ExR), inexorably leads to naïve realism and from there to metaphysical disjunctivism and its rejection of (SubC). The best way to escape the dilemma that I could find characterizes hallucination as a kind of malfunctioning perception or as an exercise of perceptual capacities, and thus perception (or the exercise of perceptual capacities) as the needed common factor. I have argued that this would not do because it either has the implausible consequence that perceived worldly facts cannot be excellent epistemic reasons. Or, on a different way of conceiving the escape route—where perceived facts are the excellent reasons—the commonality between perception and hallucination is so insubstantial that metaphysical disjunctivists can accept it after all.

ACKNOWLEDGMENTS

I would like to thank audiences at the conference on *Searle on Perception*, Bochum 2016, and at the workshop *Thinking about Perception*, Zurich 2016, particularly Mike Beaton, Nadja El Kassar, Chris Ranalli, and Charles Travis, for extremely helpful suggestions on earlier drafts of this paper. I thank David McGraw for prompting me to address the issue of object-dependent senses in a more convincing way.

REFERENCES

Byrne, A., Logue, H., 2008. Either/or. In: Haddock, A., Macpherson, F. (Eds.), Disjunctivism: Perception, Action, Knowledge. Oxford University Press, Oxford, pp. 57–93.

Cunningham, J., 2016. Reflective epistemological disjunctivism. Episteme 13, 111–132.

Dancy, J., 2000. Practical Reality. Oxford University Press, Oxford.

Evans, G., 1982. The Varieties of Reference. Clarendon Press, Oxford.

Fish, W., 2009. Perception, Hallucination, and Illusion. Oxford University Press, New York.

Frege, G., 1980. Philosophical and Mathematical Correspondence. In: Gabriel, G., et al. (Ed.). Basil Blackwell, Oxford.

Haddock, A., 2013. The disjunctive conception of perceiving. In: Willaschek, M. (Ed.), Disjunctivism: Disjunctive Accounts in Epistemology and in the Philosophy of Perception. Routledge, London, pp. 103–122.

Haddock, A., Macpherson, F., 2008. Introduction: varieties of disjunctivism. In: Disjunctivism: Perception, Action, Knowledge. Oxford University Press, Oxford, pp. 1–24.

Harman, G., 1990. The intrinsic quality of experience. In: Tomberlin (Ed.), Action Theory and Philosophy of Mind. Philosophical Perspectives, vol. 4. Ridgeview Publishing, Atascadero, CA, pp. 31–52.

Hinton, J.M., 1967/2009. Visual experiences. In: Byrne, A., Logue, H. (Eds.), Disjunctivism: Contemporary Readings. MIT Press, Cambridge, MA, pp. 1–11.

Hornsby, J., 2008. A disjunctive conception of acting for reasons. In: Haddock, A., Macpherson, F. (Eds.), Disjunctivism: Perception, Action, Knowledge. Oxford University Press, Oxford, pp. 244–261.

Johnston, M., 2004/2009. The obscure object of hallucination. In: Byrne, A., Logue, H. (Eds.), Disjunctivism: Contemporary Readings. MIT Press, Cambridge, MA, pp. 207–270.

Littlejohn, C., 2016. Pritchard's reasons. J. Philos. Res. 41, 201–219.

Logue, H., 2012. What should the naïve realist say about total hallucinations? Philos. Perspect. 26, 173–199.

Martin, M.G.F., 2004. The limits of self-awareness. Philos. Stud. 120, 37–89.

McDowell, J., 1982/2009. Criteria, defeasibility, and knowledge. In: Byrne, A., Logue, H. (Eds.), Disjunctivism: Contemporary Readings. MIT Press, Cambridge, MA, pp. 75–85.

McDowell, J., 1984. De Re senses. Philos. Q. 34, 283–294.

McDowell, J., 1994. Mind and World. Harvard University Press, Cambridge, MA.

McDowell, J., 1986/1998. Singular thought and the extent of 'inner space'. In: Meaning, Knowledge, and Reality. Harvard University Press, Cambridge, MA, pp. 228–259.

McDowell, J., 2008. The disjunctive conception of experience as material for a transcendental argument. In: Haddock, A., Macpherson, F. (Eds.), Disjunctivism: Perception, Action, Knowledge. Oxford University Press, Oxford, pp. 376–388.

McDowell, J., 2011. Perception as a Capacity for Knowledge (Aquinas Lecture). Marquette University Press, Milwaukee.

McDowell, J., 2013. Perceptual experience: both relational and contentful. Eur. J. Philos. 21, 144–157.

Moore, G.E., 1965. The refutation of idealism. In: Philosophical Studies. Routledge & Kegan Paul, London, pp. 1–30.

Pritchard, D., 2011. Evidentialism, internalism, disjunctivism. In: Dougherty, T. (Ed.), Evidentialism and Its Discontents. Oxford University Press, New York, pp. 235–253.

Pritchard, D., 2012. Epistemological Disjunctivism. Oxford University Press, Oxford.

Rödl, S., 2010. The self-conscious power of sensory knowledge. Grazer Philos. Stud. 81, 135–151.

Searle, J., 2015. Seeing Things as They Are: A Theory of Perception. Oxford University Press, New York.

Schmidt, E., 2015. Modest Nonconceptualism: Epistemology, Phenomenology, and Content. Springer, Cham.

Snowdon, P., 2005. The formulation of disjuncitivism: a response to fish. Proc. Aristot. Soc. 105, 129–141.

Sosa, D., 2011. Perceptual knowledge. In: Bernecker, S., Pritchard, D. (Eds.), The Routledge Companion to Epistemology. Routledge, London, pp. 294–304.

Soteriou, M., 2014. The disjunctive theory of perception. In: Zalta, E.N. (Ed.), The Stanford Encyclopedia of Philosophy, Summer 2014 ed. URL: http://plato.stanford.edu/ archives/sum2014/entries/perception-disjunctive/.

Tye, M., 2000. Consciousness, Color, and Content. MIT Press, Cambridge, MA.

Tye, M., 2009. Consciousness Revisited: Materialism without Phenomenal Concepts. MIT Press, Cambridge, MA.

Williamson, T., 2000. Knowledge and its Limits. Oxford University Press, Oxford.

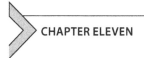

CHAPTER ELEVEN

Seeing Things: Defending Direct Perception

Fred Adams[1], Gary Fuller[2], Murray Clarke[3]
[1]Linguistics & Cognitive Science and Philosophy, University of Delaware, Newark, DE, United States;
[2]Philosophy, Central Michigan University, Mt. Pleasant, MI, United States; [3]Philosophy, Concordia University,
Montreal, Canada

1. INTRODUCTION

We think of perception (such as visual perception) as a relation between internal mental events and external physical objects. The internal mental events are not the objects of perception but the perceivings of those external objects. The objects of perception are the physical objects and events in the world around us. For the purposes of this paper, we will outline the basic tenets of this view and reply to the reasons that Robert French advances to reject the view. We shall also consider some of what we find problematic with French's defense of his own position—representative realism, a form of indirect perception.

2. DIRECT PERCEPTION

We are defending direct perception but not exactly Gibson's (1979) version. We accept that there are internal representations, but that they constitute one part of the perceptual relation to distal perceptual objects.

Consider tactile perception. Matt places his fingers on the keypad of his laptop. There is a familiar smooth feel of the surface properties of the keys. In some cases (for some keys) there are raised marks on the keys (marks that can be used to orient fingers on the keyboard, on the *F* key and the *J* key, for instance). Matt's tactile perception consists of this relation between the external source of his perceptual experiences (the keys on the keypad itself) and the internal mental perceivings that constitute Matt's part of the perceptual relation (what it *feels like* to Matt when touching the keypad). Similar cases include the Braille marks in an elevator.

The tactile perceptual episode on the mental side of the relation consists of the phenomenal qualitative feel of the keys on the keypad. At the other

Direct versus Indirect Realism
ISBN 978-0-12-812141-2
https://doi.org/10.1016/B978-0-12-812141-2.00011-8

163

end of the relation is the physical keypad itself and the properties detectable by the sensory mechanisms of the human body (via touch receptors in the fingers and nerve fibers in the hands and arms and nervous system that extends to the haptic areas of the brain where such signals from touch receptors are received). Hence, touch perception (as is all perception) is constituted by such a relation between the mental events in the head and the physical sources of perception, which are in the world (normally beyond the body—except when the body itself is being perceived).

The perceptual experience for Matt begins when the keyboard *feels some way to Matt.* There must be some discriminable difference between the mental state just prior to the perceiving of the keyboard and the beginning events of the perceiving. Tactilely it must feel differently to Matt when he is experiencing the keypad from just before the perceiving begins. Matt must be able to discriminate the difference between the nonperceptual experiential episode just prior to touching the keys and the perceptual episode that begins with the touching of the keys (Dretske, 1969).

These perceptual experiences have qualitative properties (the so-called "qualia") of the experiences. These are produced by the objects being experienced and derive their qualities from the physical qualities of the objects perceived. The qualia are produced via mental representations of the physical properties of the objects that the fingers contact. These perceptual events are representational events. The qualitative properties of the perceptual mental events are due to the physical properties represented by the mind/brain during the perceptual process. For instance, the keys feel smooth because they are smooth given the blunt instruments constituted by the touch receptors in human fingers. Finer instruments might detect less smooth surfaces. The bumps on the *F* and *J* keys are easily detected by the human touch receptors and represented as bumps because slightly raised above the rest of the surface of the keys.

We accept the so-called representational account of qualitative experience (Dretske, 1995; Tye, 1995, 2009). On this view, qualitative states of mind are representations. When of external objects, the qualitative states of mind arise because various areas of the brain have been recruited to represent types of external properties of objects and events. The sound of middle *C* on the piano as experienced is an auditory state that represents the vibrations of the strings when that note is struck. The smell of smoke is an olfactory representation of the carbon molecules in the air given off by the fire. There are neurochemical events in the brain when experiencing qualitative properties of objects and events. Yet the qualia of the experience are not solely due to the neurochemical properties in the brain, but rather to these neural properties and activations standing in a representational relationship to their external causes. The experiences are not of or about the neural events themselves, but rather are of or about the distal causes of the experiences. So the qualitative experience of the feel of keypad represents the surface properties of the keypad not an internal phenomenal state.

While we will not be concerned here with the epistemic and semantic properties of perception, we agree with Fodor and Pylyshyn (2015, Ch. 4) that the causal perceptual relation is the basis for semantic reference. Matt's tactile experiences are *about* the keys that he is perceiving and this allows him to think about and form beliefs about them, as well. In a manner reminiscent of rejection of the descriptional theory of meaning, they say perceptual object representation is of the form "this" or "that," and not as things that "fit certain descriptions" (Fodor and Pylyshyn, 2015, p. 115).

Of course, on our view this means that qualia are not reducible to the neural chemical properties of neural events alone because they are representations. Representations are of/about things and this is not merely a neurochemical matter. And what is more since qualia are representations of the properties of external objects, the view has to account for how representations can represent something at the distal end of a causal chain. This latter challenge will be directly relevant to answering some of the challenges to direct perception—some of which are offered by French and to which we will reply below. In addition, on this view (our view) it will follow that the qualitative properties of experiences do not represent themselves. Why this is important will become clear when we discuss French's solution to the "regress problem."

3. PERCEIVING DISTAL OBJECTS ACROSS CAUSAL CHAINS

When Matt experiences the keyboard, there is a causal chain that runs from the touch receptors in his fingers to the haptic areas of the brain that receive signals from the fingers. One problem for direct perception is how one's experience can be directly of the distal object in this causal chain, viz. the keyboard. How does perception jump across all the links in causal chain? Matt perceives the distal objects (the surfaces of the keys), not the events in haptic processing areas of his brain. But how?

The causal chains that produce perceptual experiences are over multiple channels (nerve pathways). To get an experience to represent a distal cause it must be the case that it is best correlated with the distal object. If a perception is a relation, then if the correlation of the relata is best coordinated between the experience and distal cause, this is why the experience represents the distal cause and not the more proximal causes. This is what some (Dretske, 1981) call giving the distal cause "primary" representation. French says he thinks Dretske's solution to the causal chain problem is the best he has seen. French says: "The clearest treatment of this topic, which I have seen is that given by Dretske (1981), which provides an analysis in terms of information theory, whereby the object of perception is identified with the object given 'primary representation' by a perceiver."

Matt's fingers have multiple nerve receptors. Each is sending a signal to the haptic areas of the brain. These areas are using this information to produce a representation of the surfaces of the keypad. The notion of "primary representation," is that though there are differences in the signals being sent along the circuits of the receptors, those signals cannot be what is represented by the brain.

In an example of auditory perception, Dretske (1981, p. 160) explains why one hears the doorbell ring, not the button being depressed, even though both pieces of information arrive at the subject. He says it is because the subject gives "primary representation" to the bell not the button. This occurs when the experience representing G (button's being depressed) depends upon the information about B (the bell's ringing), but not *vice versa*. He says: "Our auditory experience represents the bell ringing and it represents the buttons' being depressed. But only the former is given primary representation because the information the experience carries about the depression of the button depends on the informational link between the button and the bell, while its representation of the bell's ringing does not depend on this relationship."

More relevant to our view that perceptual experiences represent the distal physical objects and not the signals sent through the nerve receptors or resulting retinal images, is Dretske's example of seeing a round object. "Since the proximal (peripheral, neural) antecedents of an experience are not represented at all, they are not given primary representation.... The visual representation of a round object (its looking round) carries information about the shape of the object without carrying information about the shape of the image projected on the retina...[since]... the retinal projection is constantly changing" (Dretske, 1981, p. 163).

Though there are differences in the signals being sent along the circuits of the receptors, these signals are not what is primarily represented by the brain.

The receptors are not primarily represented because there are differences among the various signals and pathways. The only nonequivocal signal being sent is the information about the surface of the keys. The qualia of the experience will represent the distal cause (surface of the keypad) when best correlated with properties of the distal cause, not the properties of the more proximal causes. For most of us, most of the time, the information that there are signals being sent up the causal pathways actually depends on representing the surfaces of the keys (via their feels). It is not the other way around. We do not experience the keys via experiencing the way it feels for nerve endings in the fingers to be stimulated (though they are stimulated). It may be possible (perhaps when one's arm "falls asleep" or under the influence of certain kinds of drugs—lysergic acid diethylamine) to experience the nerve firings and give them primary representation, but this is not the case when Matt is in normal states and using his computer.

4. THE REGRESS PROBLEM

The generalized regress problem is something any theory of perception must face. In the causal chain from distal object to perceiving subject, there will be representations of the distal object. The regress problem arises in dealing with the utilization of the internal representations of the distal object. Were one to posit a mechanism of perception of the internal representation similar to the mechanism for representing the distal object itself, the regress is launched. So, to avoid the regress one must explain how the internal representation of the distal object is utilized by the brain without launching the regress.

Think first of simple mechanisms that use representing structures. The thermostat represents the temperature in the room and the set point for turning on the furnace. These are natural representations of temperature and desired temperature. When the room temperature drops below the set point the circuit closes (representing the room temperature's dropping below the desired temperature). Utilization of this representation is simply the circuit's closing and sending a signal to the furnace. There is no need of something to *read* the representation. The system is designed by the heating engineer in such a way that the internal structures, which constitute the internal representation do their job without needing to themselves, be represented further.

In the case of Matt perceiving the keypad, there are internal representations that have phenomenal content, unlike the thermostat. So one might think that this makes matters significantly different, opening the door for a regress. But this is not so. The internal states, which have phenomenal content, are the representations of the distal object (in this case, the keypad). When Matt feels the keys, his brain's utilization of these phenomenal representations is to cause beliefs, to cause motor activity in his brain that constitutes the signals to his fingers to type. Just as in the case of the simple thermostat, there is no need of further representations to represent his perceptions of the keypad.

Having phenomenal content is a matter of the haptic system being recruited to fire selectively with respect to the features of the keypad, recruited to represent properties that can be discriminated haptically. This would include solidity, shape, smoothness, bumps on homing keys, and so on. These cause in Matt the corresponding qualitative feels when typing. The brain's utilization of these perceptual representations works in tandem with his intentions—what he is intending to do when his phenomenal states feel thus and thus (the way they feel when typing). Even when there are phenomenal states involved, the neural system is designed in such a way to utilize these representations straight away without need for further haptic representations of the haptic representations of the keypad.

Hence there is no regress in the perceptual causal chain.

Of course, Matt is capable of having beliefs and desires and conscious awareness of his phenomenal states. But these are epistemic states and involve epistemic access to his perceptual states. These are not themselves in the direct causal chain between distal object and perceptual state that constitute the relation of directly perceiving the keypad (Smith, 2002). In fact, almost all cases, there are modular noncognitively penetrable perceptual states (Pylyshyn, 1999). For example, though we know the Müller-Lyer lines are the same length, we cannot change the fact that they look to be of different lengths.

5. ROBERT FRENCH'S REASONS FOR THE REJECTION OF DIRECT PERCEPTION

Before we begin, we should point out that French distinguishes two forms of perception: an epistemic form and an ontic form.

The epistemic form involves states such as seeing as, seeing that. In these states, concepts are involved. Another way of making perception epistemic according to French is when inferences are involved in the perceptual process.

On the ontic version, perception is nonepistemic (Dretske, 1969, 2000). In this case, experiences of seeing do not involve concepts or inferences. In a case of nonepistemic or ontic perception, one may see an X but not see it as an X. Indeed, one need not apply any concept at all to an object X to have a visual experience of X. But one would neither know it was an X nor would have any inference about its being an X, nor any inference involved in its being a visual experience of X. An infant in its crib might well see the mobile above its head without *seeing* it or any of its parts *as* the objects that they are.

French limits his objections to direct perception to the ontic versions of perception. So we will not discuss his remarks about epistemic perception, except when discussing his account of the theory-laden nature of perception–language.

French's first reason for rejecting direct perception is the argument from illusion. He does not actually lay out the argument but mentions things such as the Ames room illusions, rotating trapezoid illusions, and the fact that three-dimensional (3D) movie experiences are produced via two-dimensional (2D) stimuli.

The argument from illusion has the following form. We will start with visual illusions, but the arguments could use any sensory modality. S experiences X, but the distal object is not X, so S cannot be experiencing the distal object X. A common example is Jill seeing the stick in the water. The stick appears to be bent. But the stick is not actually bent. So what Jill sees (what appears to her) cannot be the actual stick.

The mistake in the argument from illusion is the move from the fact that the stick appears bent to there being something that is bent that Jill sees. Whereas, in fact there is nothing that is bent that Jill sees. She sees the stick. The appearance of its being bent is caused by the refraction of light through the medium of water. Straight sticks appear bent when placed in water. So what Jill sees is the straight stick appearing bent due to the refraction of light, which is mediating the perceptual relation between Jill and the straight stick. So it is mistake to think that the argument from illusion is a good reason to reject direct perception.

The Ames room illusion is very similar. Suppose when looking into the room Peg sees Alice who appears to be the same size as the normal coffee cup also in the room. The argument says since Peg is seeing a cup and Alice that are of the same height and since Alice and the cup are not actually the same size, Peg cannot be seeing the actual cup and the actual Alice. Instead, the argument suggests that Peg must be seeing a phenomenal Alice and a phenomenal cup. According to the argument, Peg sees two objects that are of the same height. But the actual objects, Alice and the cup, are not of the same height. So, Peg cannot be seeing the actual objects and instead must be seeing a phenomenal Alice and a phenomenal cup.

But the same mistake recurs. It does not follow from the fact that Alice and cup appear the same size that there are things the same size that Peg is seeing. What is really going on is that Peg is seeing the actual cup and the actual Alice, but because of the construction of the room it produces visual cues from the objects in the room that distort the appearance of the actual objects Peg sees. The perceptual relation between Peg's visual experiences and the distal objects in the room is mediated by the light coming from the actual objects in the Ames room. Given the distorted cues, Alice and cup appear the same size. Nonetheless, it is the actual Alice and actual cup that Peg sees directly. There are no phenomenal perceptual objects in Peg's visual experience spatially between Peg's experiences and Alice and the cup. It also does not follow from the fact that Peg's experiences incorrectly represent the size of Alice and the cup that Peg's experiences correctly represent some phenomenal objects in between Peg and the distal objects. There are no direct perceptions of such phenomenal objects because there are no such phenomenal objects. There are internal states with phenomenal content, but these representational states do not represent themselves.

Fodor & Pylyshyn agree with us on these matters. Here is how Fodor and Pylyshyn (2015, pp. 113–114) describe the Ames room: "…a distorted room with no actual rectangular surfaces, constructed in such a way that the projection of every line and polygon in the room onto the retina of an observer looking through a peephole is identical to the projection that would arise from an actual 3D room with walls at right angles to each other and to the floor and ceiling…it is possible to build because there are many ways to build a 3D object that projects onto a given 2D pattern—the 3D-to-2D mapping is many-to-one."

Unlike French who we presume thinks there are inferences at work in such illusions, we agree with Fodor and Pylyshyn who respond to such illusions saying: "…despite inherent ambiguity of the 2D image can be explained without having to assume that the visual system draws inferences from specific knowledge regarding what a particular 3D scene is likely to contain…. The visual system is so constructed, presumably because it has become tuned over eons of evolutionary history so that the possible inter-pretations it is able to make are severely restricted."

While French does not include arguments from hallucination, we will explain why they too do not refute direct perception. The general form of an argument from hallucination is the following: *S* perceives *Y* but there is no distal object *Y*, so *S* must be perceiving a phenomenal object *Y*. While experiencing delirium tremens (DTs) the alcoholic "sees snakes," but there are no snakes. Therefore, what the alcoholic sees cannot be actual distal objects. But he sees something, so he must be seeing some phenomenal object (phenomenal snake).

The proper rejection of the argument from hallucination is that when the alcoholic hallucinates snakes, he sees nothing. Not an actual distal snake but not a phenomenal snake either. True, something in his body may be stimulating his visual receptors as they would be stimulated where he observing snakes. This accounts for the snakelike appearances caused by his detoxification. But there are no objects being perceived (distal or phenomenal).

Since, on our view, perception is a relation between the experience in the head and the distal object in the world, it is possible for a veridical and nonveridical experience to be qualitatively the same. However, it does not follow from this that one is not directly perceiving something when there is a distal object. It does not follow because perception involves a *relation* between what is in the head and what is in the world under the proper conditions for that relation to support veridicality. So detoxing Rob and nondetoxing Rob have qualitatively similar experiences of snakes but only nondetoxing Rob is actually seeing something (i.e., snakes).

Another mistake, we think we see French make, is to construct a mistaken dilemma that either Naïve Realism is true or Indirect Perception is true. Then he gives reasons for thinking Naïve Realism is false and wants to draw the conclusion that Indirect Perception follows. But not all direct perception theorists must accept Naïve Realism. The direct perception theorist can accept that perceptual experiences can distort reality. According to French, the Naïve Realist would have to accept that the world really is the way it is immediately presented. So if the stick looks bent, it must really be bent. Since it is not really bent, the Naïve view is false. But we can reject such a Naïve view, without rejecting direct perception (as we do above in defending against the arguments from illusion and hallucination).

French's second objection to direct perception is the argument from causal chains. He seems to hold that the presence of intervening causal processes between distal object and perceiver implies that direct perception is false (French, pp. 6–7). Our discussion earlier of how a distal object can be *primarily represented* across a causal chain shows that French is wrong here. Since we gave our solution to the worry above, we will not replay it now. Suffice it to say that any account of direct perception must explain how perception can traverse the causal chains that mediate perception. We have explained it in terms of perception being a relation between perceiver and perceived. And the perceiver perceives the distal object when that object is best correlated (in terms of information and representation) with the distal object.

French's third reason to reject direct perception is a curious rejection of what he sees as ordinary language's bias toward direct perception. After giving hints that ordinary language (Austin, 1962; Ryle, 1949) may favor direct perception, French claims that a proper reconstruction of language will favor his indirect perception (representational realism).

Why does French think ordinary languages favor direct perception? French cites examples where perception terms are success (achievement) terms: "'see' is what Ryle called an 'achievement word' in the sense that its correct application presupposes the existence of the object, which it is being claimed is being seen." He continues: "…when we claim to see an object, we claim to be immediately…aware of at least a portion of the object, although we do not have to be aware of each part of the complete object…." He also says: "…we also hold that what we see here is physical, and that it continues to exist in the same format when nobody is looking at it" (French, p. 11).

French is talking about *claims to see.* Within the context of *claims* perception terms need not be achievement terms. Contrast touch. If Gary touches the cup, there must be a cup. This is not about what Gary claims. It is about a physical relation between Gary and the cup. Contrast that with the claim Rob makes, while going through DTs. Rob claims to see a cup, but there is no cup. Rob did not misuse the term "see." So the logic of *claims to see* is different from the use of the term "see."

It is a mistake to run together matters about *seeing* with matters about *claims to see.*

What is more, when detoxing Rob utters: "I see snakes," it does not follow that there are snakes. And again, Rob is not misspeaking.

We take it that what French meant to say is that "seeing" as ordinarily used is an achievement (success) term. If "Gary sees the cup" is true, then there will be a cup. The truth conditions for the sentence require the existence of the cup. French clearly wants to add that if it is true that Gary sees the cup, then the cup is a physical object that continues to exist when no one is looking. But these are not sufficient for direct realism. Bishop Berkeley could make the same first claim and the second (because Berkeley reinterprets "physical object"). Or, if one sees Murray in the mirror via seeing a mirror image of Murray, Murray will be there. In this case, seeing him is quite indirect (on our view). We have no problem with some cases of indirect perception where both the directly and indirectly perceived objects are physical. Another example of such a case would be that of indirectly perceiving a car in virtue of directly perceiving the front of the car. So even if "see" is an achievement term, it is neutral between direct and indirect perception or realism *versus* idealism.

Why does French think a reconstruction of language is needed in science?

As far as we can tell only because he needs this to be the case for his view to be true. We have explained why ordinary language is neutral. He gives no reasons, based on science, to think a rational reconstruction of language is required. He does give examples from science where ordinary terms have been made more precise, but he does not give reasons from science why *perception terms* must rationally reconstructed. He gives no examples where perception scientists are compelled to rationally reconstruct perception terms.

The one example he does give that is relevant is about color terms. But the philosophical debate still rages over whether colors are objectively real. One cannot appeal to color science (yet) to support direct or indirect perception without begging the question of whether perception is direct or indirect.

6. ROBERT FRENCH'S OWN SOLUTION TO THE REGRESS PROBLEM

The regress problem is that in the causal chain of perception there will be the following: the distal object perceived, and the internal mental events that constitute the representation of the distal object. But to utilize the internal representation of the distal object, there must be a perceiving subject who experiences the internal representation. However, if there is an experiencing subject experiencing the internal representation of the distal object, there must be another experiencing subject capable of experiencing the internal representation. This requires a new internal representation within the experiencing subject. However, this causal chain is replicated indefinitely, and one has a regress.

French thinks objections can be raised to his indirect realism based on a regress argument. In fact, he has three versions of the regress argument (involving multiple internal "eyes," internal homunculi, and sense data). In the case of multiple eyes, there would have to be an internal set of eyes to experience the internal representation of the distal object, and then one is off and running along the chain of the regress, constituting a problem for any theory of perception, including French's.

French's solution to the regress problem begins by talking about the function of the eye. After discussing the function of the eye, he asks the question of "…why, once such a focusing operation has been performed in the visual perception process, there should be any need to have it be repeated at a later stage, as was implied by the claim that further eyes, as optical systems, would be required…?"

French is responding to Gibson (1950), who, in his polemic, suggested that there must be a second eye to perceive the picture created by the retinal image in the process of perception. French's reply is that, once the function of the first eye is complete, there is no need for a second eye to perceive the retinal image. He recounts specific functions that parts of the visual system perform in response to specific stimuli. Hence, French's reply to the "multiple eye" version is simply to say that only one eye is required once we understand how the eye works.

However, Gibson's polemic seems to suggest that the reason a second eye is needed is to perceive the representation created via the retinal image. Merely focusing on specificity of how the eye works, does not properly address Gibson's charge. To answer Gibson, one must explain why no eye is required to process the information contained in the representation caused by the retinal image, not merely to tell us how the one eye we have works.

The closest he comes to answering Gibson's polemic is when he denies a regress of homunculi. But once again the reply is in terms of the specific details of how the eye works. However, once we understand the specifics of how the eye works, the problem is to explain what the brain does with the information supplied by the eye. French seems to think that once we know everything about how the eye works, we will know all we need to know about how the brain uses information supplied by the retinal image.

If indirect realism (French's representational realism) is true, we perceive something like a picture of the distal object. But if we perceive something like a picture, then one seems to need another eye to perceive the picture of the distal stimulus. Merely denying that there is another eye leaves unexplained how the internal picture (representation) is utilized by the brain or how it is the real object of perception. French's view requires that what one perceives (since not the distal object) is the inner phenomenal object. But if one accepts that there is another mechanism of perception (maybe not involving an actual eye), one still needs an account of what happens when the brain perceives the proximal representation (not the distal object). Perhaps there is literally no "eye," but he still owes us an explanation of what constitutes *the perceiving act* on his account of indirect or "representational" realism.

One might fall back on a homuncular version of perception, where a homunculus is involved in the perceiving of the proximal representation. But French also rejects the homuncular account. How does he reject the homucular account? By telling us more about the specific functions of the eye. However, that will not do. It will not do unless the functions of the eye alone constitute the act of indirectly perceiving the proximal object of perceptions. But of course the perceptual areas of the brain are involved in the act of perceiving, and French seems not even indirectly to gesture in that direction in his solution to the regress problem. Knowing everything there is to be known about how the eye works will not alone solve the regress problem. One needs to know how the perceptual areas of the brain utilize the information being sent from the brain. One needs to know how the qualitative states of the visual brain come to represent and how they cause things in virtue of being the representations that they are. French seems to have nothing to say about this.

The third type of the regress argument (Ryle, 1949) suggests that when one has a visual representation there is an internal sense datum. Then having that sense datum again requires a further sensing and sense datum. French seems to think that the way out of this regress argument depends on the theory-laden properties of language. We have responded to this above. We doubt seriously that regimenting language solves such problems as regress arguments.

One last point: French needs an account where the regress stops when the perceiving of the proximal representation and the proximal representation's representing the distal object collapse. That is, the way out of the regress demands that there is no further eye, and no further homunculus, and yet perception is still indirect. So the object of perception must be some internal object, and the perceiving of that internal object must be identical with that internal object perceived. "The very existence of sense data, in as much as it is a phenomenal existence, constitutes their being sensed. Thus, it is also held that the distinction between the 'sensor' and the 'sensed' breaks down (French, p. 6)." Otherwise, we could recreate the regress. So, it looks to us as though French is stuck with internal mental representations that represent themselves.

An ordinary picture of a dog partly consists of a photographic surface filled with 2D figures, but it is not also a picture of those 2D figures. It is a picture of a 3D dog. Usually, representations do not represent themselves. Perhaps the linguistic and conceptual representation "This sentence is short" is an exception. But on French's view that is what is directly represented—phenomenal objects. All such phenomenal representations would have to represent themselves (to stop the regress). This consequence surely is absurd.

7. CONCLUSION

In this paper, we have sketched an account of direct perception. We have explained that perception is a relation between perceiving subject and distal object mediated by phenomenal experiences. We have not gone into matter such as blindsight, which involves perceptual relations but not necessarily conscious phenomenal experiences. Nonetheless, blindsight would not threaten direct perception.

We have explained how to account for several challenges to direct perception. We mainly addressed those raised by French, but his objections are not uncommon in the literature on perception. We explained how to handle the arguments from illusion and hallucination, and regress, and we explained how perception can traverse the links in the causal chain of perception.

We then turned our attention to French's reasons for accepting indirect perception (which he calls "representational realism"). We dismissed his reasons against direct perception and found fault with his own attempt to explain away the regress problem. We denied his claim that ordinary language is biased toward Naïve Realism and suggested that rational reconstructions of language must be driven by scientific reasons, if at all.

We are very pleased to have been included in this project and thank the editor and publishers of the volume for our inclusion. We also thank our good friend Mordecai for support and encouragement during the writing of this chapter.

REFERENCES

Austin, J.L., 1962. Sense and Sensibilia. Oxford University Press, Oxford.

Dretske, F.I., 1969. Seeing and Knowing. University of Chicago Press, Chicago.

Dretske, F., 1981. Knowledge and the Flow of Information. MIT/Bradford, Cambridge, MA.

Dretske, F., 1995. Naturalizing the Mind. MIT/Bradford, Cambridge, MA.

Dretske, F., 2000. Simple seeing. In: Perception, Knowledge and Belief. Cambridge University Press, Cambridge, UK, pp. 97–112.

Fodor, J.A., Pylyshyn, Z.W., 2015. Minds Without Meanings. MIT Press, Cambridge, MA.

French, R. A Defense of Representational Realism. In: French, R. (Ed.), Direct versus Indirect Realism: A Neurophilosophical Debate on Consciousness, Elsevier, Brooklyn.

Gibson, J.J., 1950. The Perception of the Visual World. Houghton Mifflin, Boston.

Gibson, J.J., 1979. The Ecological Approach to Visual Perception. Houghton Mifflin, Boston.

Pylyshyn, Z.W., 1999. Is vision continuous with cognition? The case for cognitive impenetrability of visual perception. Behav. Brain Sci. 22 (3), 341–423.

Ryle, G., 1949. The Concept of Mind. Hutchinson & Co, London.

Smith, A.D., 2002. The Problem of Perception. Harvard University Press, Cambridge, MA.

Tye, M., 1995. Ten Problems of Consciousness. MIT Press, Cambridge, MA.

Tye, M., 2009. Consciousness Revisited. MIT/Bradford, Cambridge, MA.

PART THREE

The Debate

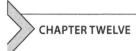

CHAPTER TWELVE

Critiques of Papers by Indirect Realists by Direct Realists

Robert French
Adjunct Instructor, Philosophy, Oakland Community College, Waterford Township, MI, United States

EVA SCHMIDT'S COMMENTS ON ROBERT FRENCH, "A DEFENSE OF REPRESENTATIONAL REALISM"

In his contribution to this anthology, Robert French defends a version of indirect realism, which he calls "representational realism", against several objections. I will here comment on French's responses (1) to the regress objection, (2) to the objection that perception is manifestly direct, and (3) to the objection from ordinary language.

1. Ryle (1949) argues that, if we understand S's perception of an ordinary physical object via her sensing of a purely mental *sensum*, we end up with an infinite regress. For we will have to understand S's sensing of this *sensum* in terms of her sensing another *sensum*, and so on. French (p. 6) responds to this by arguing that the alleged regress arises from the fact that our ordinary perception verbs (such as "perceive," "sense") are transitive. They suggest that there is a distinction between the perceiver and what she perceives. Later on (p. 37) he argues that we need to rationally reconstruct our ordinary language to allow for a phenomenal variant of perception verbs—corresponding to our sensing of percepts—which is not transitive.

I disagree with French both on the point that the feature of perception verbs of being transitive is to blame for the apparent regress, and on the point that introducing intransitive perception verbs for percepts has a bearing on the regress problem. That verbs such as "perceive" or "sense" are transitive means that they take an object. For instance, we might say that Miyumi senses the heat of the fire, or that Oscar senses a red and round sense datum. But this way of talking is not what is at the bottom of the regress. The regress, I believe, is due to the fact that perceiving an ordinary physical thing is taken, by Ryle, to be the same kind of perceptual relation as sensing a percept. Given this, if the former relation needs to be understood in terms of a further sensing relation, then the same is true for the latter relation.

Direct versus Indirect Realism
ISBN 978-0-12-812141-2
https://doi.org/10.1016/B978-0-12-812141-2.00012-X

But why should the representational realist accept that they are the same kind of relation? It seems natural to say that the perceptual relation between me and a thing in the external world requires a completely different account than the relation between me and the content of my awareness, understood as the thing that is currently on my mind. It seems that the burden of proof is on French's opponent to show that just because ordinary perceiving is a relation to an object, as is sensing, it is both times the same kind of relation.

Secondly, I am not convinced by French's attempt to get rid of the appearance of a regress by introducing intransitive "sensing" locutions. An example he gives (p. 37) is "an active voice equivalent to the passive voice 'redness is sensed (or apprehended) in a particular location in my phenomenal perceptual field.'" The idea is that this locution drops the distinction between the senser and what is sensed, so that we are not moved to account for yet another relation of someone's sensing something.

My worry here is that this rephrasing makes no difference to the regress threat. If there are phenomenal features that are sensed in someone's perceptual field, the fact of the matter is that there is a subject, that the subject has a perceptual field, and that the perceptual field includes certain sensible features. If so, there will be some or other relation between the subject, her perceptual field, and the included features. Even if French were to adopt something like a qualia view of perceptual experience, which rejects an act/object distinction between sensing and percept, we can still ask how the subject, her perceptual experiences, and their qualitative features are related. We can expect that the relation will turn out to be quite different from that between a perceiver and a perceived worldly object.

This indeed removes the regress threat. Note, however, that what is doing the work now is not how we talk, but the representational realist's insistence that the sensing relation and the perceiving relation are simply different; which is, as I have argued, the way one should respond to the regress objection in the first place.

2. French discusses the worry that a representational realist cannot allow that perception is direct, i.e., puts us in immediate touch with our surroundings, even though it manifestly does. In response, he distinguishes two senses of "direct." The first (epistemic) sense incorporates the idea that perception is noninferential and results in the claim that the percept involved in a perceptual state is qualitatively identical with the

perceived worldly object. The second (ontological) sense involves the idea that there are no causal intermediaries between percept and perceived worldly object. According to this reading, percept and perceived worldly object must be numerically identical. French concedes that representational realism cannot make room for directness in the second ontological sense (which he finds problematic anyway), but argues that the view is at least not committed to denying epistemic directness.

I want to point out here that there is a third sense of "direct," viz. that what is present to our consciousness in perception, or partly constitutes its subjective character, is the worldly objects (and the properties they instantiate) themselves. This seems to be what naïve realists and direct realists more generally have in mind—there are no other entities such as sense data that we are really immediately aware of, and that then represent worldly objects to us. This—call it the central sense of "direct"—differs from the epistemic sense that French describes. It is concerned not with the process by which we arrive at perception but with a constitutive description of what perception involves. A direct realist can even allow that there are subpersonal analogues of inferences going on in the perceptual systems when we perceive. Even if this is the case, it is possible that the phenomenal character of perception is constituted by the things we perceive and their properties.

Moreover, the central sense of "direct" is not the same as French's ontological sense, for it does not identify the worldly thing perceived with anything, particularly not with a percept. (Admittedly, it partly grounds the conscious character of perception in features of the worldly things that are perceived. But that is not to say there is an identity between two objects, a percept and a worldly object.) On the one hand, this kind of directness allows that there is a difference between the mental state of perceiving and the thing perceived. On the other hand, it is naturally combined with a denial that there is a percept as the nonphysical immediate object of perception. So, the worldly object that is perceived cannot be identified with this alleged immediate object either. A proponent of this kind of directness of perception *can* allow that there is a percept involved in perceiving, when we take this to be a subpersonal representation, or vehicle, which underlies the subject's perceiving the worldly object. Note, however, that the representational vehicle is not what is perceived, on such a view, but is merely something that is involved in making the subject's perception of the object possible. So again, there is no need to commit on the perceived object's identity with the percept.

I believe that saving this third sense of "direct" is what direct realists are concerned with; they criticize indirect realist views for denying that perception is direct in this sense.

3. French argues that our ordinary language about perception is theory-laden in that it allows only for a physical object of perception and not for the phenomenal sense of "sense" or "perceive" that representational realism needs. It presupposes the truth of naïve realism. (p. 36) He appeals to J. L. Austin (1962), who denies that ordinary language contains two senses of "perceive." According to French's reading, Austin endorses the claim that ordinary language only ever ascribes to us that we perceive *physical* objects.

I have to disagree with French's interpretation of Austin on this last point. I think the correct way to think about him is as a pluralist about the nature of the objects of perception. Austin mocks the philosophical claim that ordinary people believe that the only things we perceive are "moderate-sized specimens of dry goods" (Austin, 1962, p. 8). Austin himself claims, by contrast:

> There is no one kind of thing that we 'perceive' but many different kinds …: pens are in many ways though not in all ways unlike rainbows, which are in many ways though not in all ways unlike after-images, which in turn are in many ways but not in all ways unlike pictures on the cinema-screen – and so on, without assignable limit.
>
> **Austin (1962, p. 4)**

A further, clearly nonphysical object that he allows that a deluded subject may experience is a mirage (Austin, 1962, p. 32). Additionally, he (1962, p. 95) holds that if a subject sees an object, this entails that the object exists—though he allows that it may not have the properties that the subject perceives it as having. Given this, Austin is clearly willing to say that rainbows, after-images, or even mirages exist, even though we ordinarily would not consider them to be material objects. He thinks that their existence is presupposed in ordinary language.

So French's interesting claim that ordinary language conflicts with the claims of representational realism does not go through if Austin is correct: Ordinary language, on Austin's view, allows that all kinds of regular or outlandish things may be perceived—the only assumption that ordinary language has trouble with is that something is seen where *nothing* exists.

So, for Austin, ordinary language is not theory-laden in the way French suggests. At the same time, Austin would certainly resist French's move to introduce two distinct senses of "sense," "perceive," or the like. This move perpetuates the picture of perception that Austin wants to resist—that we can never be said to perceive run-of-the-mill things around us, period. He tries to resist this move by making it superfluous: There is no need to introduce a way of talking about perception of sense data (or percepts) in addition to our ordinary talk about perception. For our ordinary ways of speaking about perception already perfectly cover everything that we can perceive.

EVA SCHMIDT'S COMMENTS ON JOHN SMYTHIES "THE METAPHYSICAL FOUNDATIONS OF CONTEMPORARY NEUROSCIENCE: A HOUSE BUILT ON SAND"

In his contribution, Smythies claims that the metaphysical presuppositions that neuroscientists make are seriously out of step with what we know about the constitution of the world. He discusses (1) the three-dimensionalist world view of neuroscientists, which conflicts with the result from the special theory of relativity that the universe is a four-dimensional space-time worm; (2) the direct realist conception of perception as direct contact with worldly objects, which is contradicted by what neuroscience itself has shown, viz. that the objects of perception are the products of neural processes and thus distinct from the worldly objects causing these processes; and (3) the identity theory of the mind, which cannot be correct because neural states and mental states clearly have different properties. I will here focus on the first two of Smythies's points (though I disagree with the third as well.)

As Smythies states, special relativity treats time as a dimension more or less on a par with the three spatial dimensions. He concludes from this, first, that ordinary objects are not three-dimensional, but four-dimensional, and second, that objects do not change: They are eternal, immobile things that just have different properties at different space-time locations. This comes down to a perdurantist picture of objects, according to which they are not wholly present at any one time but have temporal parts, and, moreover, to an eternalist view of time, according to which all times are equally real, as opposed to a presentist view, on which only the ever-changing "now" really exists.

The conflict with neuroscience has its source (p. 222) in the fact that it treats the brain as a three-dimensional something in which change does take place, in which events occur and can be studied by (they believe, themselves changing and moving) neuroscientists. What is really going on, according to Smythies, is that there is the four-dimensional, unchangeable block universe, including four-dimensional brain space-time worms, and additionally another type of time, the "real-time t2 in which the Observer moves" and which explains why things, including brains, appear to change to human observers. If I understand him correctly, this is a distinct, but equally real time and space. At the end of the article, he says that "[w]hat we experience is phenomenal space" and suggests that "phenomenal space and physical space are ontologically and geometrically different spaces." He thinks that this is not a problem for the everyday practice of experimental neuroscience, however.

My interpretation of these claims is that Smythies holds that, in addition to the actual four-dimensional world we inhabit, there is a phenomenal world of our own creation, which has only three spatial dimensions and, as a distinct phenomenon, temporal change. So it appears that, while neuroscientists strive to learn how the actual physical brains works, their observations are sadly limited to the workings of the phenomenal brain. Smythies does not draw out this conclusion, but it fits with his claim that we cannot point at the location of our actual brain: When we try, we instead "point […] to the head that [we] experience. This is a mistake—how can the brain be in the experienced head when the experienced head is in the brain?" (p. 27).

He thereby also rejects direct realism, the claim that we are immediately confronted with worldly objects in perception. He instead adheres to the representative theory. According to this view, what we perceive is what the brain *constructs* based on its conclusions, by inference to the best explanation, as to what is present in our environment. In support of this view, Smythies points out that color, shape, and movement are processed at different speeds, so that we do not see them all at the same time (which is what direct realists would have to claim). Further, he holds that since phantom limbs are possible, the body we perceive cannot be our physical body but must be an entity constructed in the brain.

I take issue with several of Smythies's claims and arguments.

1. *Space-time and the impossibility of movement and change*: Here, Smythies progresses much too fast. For one, the mathematical representation of time as a dimension similar to the spatial dimensions in the special theory of relativity does not automatically commit us to the picture of the universe as a four-dimensional, eternal, unchangeable block. The first is a mathematical model used in theoretical physics, the second a philosophical/metaphysical claim. This is not to deny that the two claims appear to fit together quite nicely. Nonetheless, we need an argument why the claim from theoretical physics cannot be made compatible with more

intuitive views of space, time, and ordinary objects. This is especially true seeing as (according to Smythies) the block universe view violates many of our apparently indispensable assumptions about the world—such as that there is change or that we see ordinary worldly objects directly.

For another, even if we accept that the universe is an eternal, four-dimensional block, this by itself does not exclude the possibility of change or movement or of direct perception of things in the world. We might say that an object, e.g., someone's brain, changes whenever there is a difference between the features it has at two different points along the temporal dimension. And an object moves when it is at two different spatial locations at two consecutive times. I do not see what speaks against interpreting change and movement in these ways—it seems that this just what change and movement *are*, according to this view. It is consistent with an unproblematic way of conceiving of spatial differences as a kind of change, where we can say, for instance, that the German landscape changes between the North Sea and Bavaria, as it goes from flat to hilly to mountainous. If all this is correct, there is no reason to introduce a distinct phenomenal time to account for the apparent change and movements of things.

2. *The untenability of direct realism*: Even if there is no change or movement because of how space-time is constituted, this does not defeat direct realism. As a paradigmatic version of direct realism, take intentionalism, the view that perceptual experience, just like belief, essentially represents the world as being a certain way (Tye, 1995). That is to say, it has a content, which is responsible for its phenomenal character. It is a variety of direct realism because it holds that experience *immediately* presents the subject with her surroundings, not mediated by sense data or the like. This view accounts for illusions and hallucinations by saying that they *mis*represent the subject's environment. It could therefore easily allow that our experience of movement and temporal change is a grand illusion—experience simply misrepresents the stationary, unchanging world. The same goes for our experience of the four-dimensional world as three-dimensional. But this does not mean that there is an extra phenomenal space and time. Rather the situation is exactly analogous to someone's mistakenly believing that there are only the three spatial dimensions, which does not entail that there is an extra space and time of her belief either. For the naïve realist, what counts is that we are related to worldly objects, even if we get some of their properties wrong. For a naïve realist account of illusion, see Brewer (2008).

Alternatively, an intentionalist could insist that perceptual experience represents physical objects directly, though under a three-dimensional aspect or mode of presentation. The idea might be that we only ever represent tiny cross-sections of four-dimensional objects in experience, and that we represent the temporal dimension merely by representing, consecutively, the given features of objects (and this is just what we mistakenly conceive of as change or movement). Again, there is no need to introduce an additional three-dimensional space that involves genuine temporal change.

As to the additional problems that Smythies raises for direct realism (processing of visual stimuli and phantom limb), I do not see how they are threatening at all to the view. Everyone accepts that neural processing underlies perception—it is what is needed to establish our direct perception of our surroundings. It does not seem relevant that some visible features are processed more quickly than others. For the intentionalist, the way to think about this would simply be that not all features of physical objects begin to be visually represented at the same time. The naïve realist might say that the perceptual relation between the subject and the seen object is expanded over time, first including only a relation to the object and its color, but then also to its shape and finally its motion. This seems unproblematic, for it happens in other cases as well. For instance, when I look at a slowly spinning statue, I at first perceive (visually represent/am related to) only the visible features instantiated by its front but later also to those of its sides or back.

Phantom limbs do not pose a special problem for direct realism either. They are typical examples of hallucination, and will be treated by direct realists in the normal way. Intentionalists will treat them as cases of misrepresentation, in which an object (the limb) is represented in a place where there is nothing. Naïve realists will say that, as a hallucination, it is a mental state substantially different from the indistinguishable veridical perception of the limb. (This follows from the fact that, for the naïve realist, a perception of a limb is essentially a relation to the limb, whose phenomenal character is partly constituted by the limb and its perceptible features, whereas there is no actual limb to be related to in phantom limb cases. See Martin, 2009.) Unfortunately our powers of discrimination between our perceptions and some of our hallucinations are very limited, so that subjects of phantom limb experiences mistake them for perceptions of real limbs, or so the naïve realist thinks. There is certainly more to be said about the plausibility or implausibility of either direct realist proposal; my point here is merely that the above perceptual phenomena by themselves are not very interesting obstacles. The interesting work would begin after acknowledging the intentionalist, and naïve realist accounts of these phenomena, by showing that they are somehow inadequate.

3. *The defensibility of an extra phenomenal space and time*: If Smythies is right that we only experience the phenomenal space and time that our brain constructs, there is indeed a *practical* problem for experimental neuroscience. This is not that neuroscientists use three-dimensional terminology to investigate a four-dimensional world, but rather that the experiments that neuroscientists conduce are aimed at understanding the functioning of the actual physical brain whose processing gives rise to our mental lives. But on Smythies's account, it is not clear how they are in any position at all to learn or even to talk about the brain that does this, when their experiments are allegedly limited to merely manipulating the three-dimensional world constructed by the brain. This is at the very least a practical problem. For neuroscientists would need some additional philosophical principle allowing them to draw conclusions from what they find out by experiments about their mental constructs (the brain in the brain, so to speak) to what is going on in the actual brain.

But these considerations bring out a more principled problem for Smythies's representative realism. The basic worry goes back to Berkeley (2008, p. 89/90). He argues that once we accept that all we are ever confronted with are ideas (or brain-made constructs); our knowledge of the physical objects that allegedly produce them is forfeit. In Berkeley's argument, the point is that there is not only no deductive route from ideas to material objects but also no inductive reasoning that would support claims about the makeup of the world beyond our experience, starting from our ideas.

To apply the Berkeleian point to Smythies's view: How could theorists' research that, due to what perception is limited to, takes as its evidence only entities existing in the three-dimensional phenomenal space, give us any definite results about the physical, four-dimensional world? Again, we need some principles that tell us how to bridge the gap between our phenomenal world and the physical world. These principles would need to be justified somehow. In light of this, one might worry how theoretical physicists can establish anything about the four-dimensional constitution of the physical world in the first place. I assume that physicists take themselves to theorize not about constructs created by their own brains but about the actual physical world. If they have never succeeded in doing so in the first place, there might be hope that the problem that Smythies points to does not arise at all. So there is no need to introduce a distinction between a physical, four-dimensional space and a phenomenal three-dimensional space either.

EVA SCHMIDT'S COMMENTS ON DAVID MCGRAW, "AGAINST THE COMBINATION OF MATERIALISM AND DIRECT REALISM"

In his contribution "Against the Combination of Materialism and Direct Realism," David McGraw argues that direct realism conflicts with materialism. There are fundamental differences between the phenomenal qualities of our perceptual experiences and the properties of the physical things we perceive. So the attempt to spell out the phenomenal character of perceptual experience in terms of features of the things we experience is bound to lead to trouble for a proponent of materialism.

In this comment, I will argue that there need not be any conflict between direct realism and materialism, given a proper understanding of direct realism and the replies available to the view.

McGraw holds that, when a subject sees a wall, she has a visual impression of it, in virtue of which she perceives the actual wall. He argues that the impression is numerically distinct from the wall by pointing out that the wall keeps on existing when the subject looks away and thus loses the impression. The impression is within the perceiver, according to McGraw.

The claim that there is a visual impression could be interpreted in at least two ways. On the one hand, it might be the claim that when the subject sees the wall, she undergoes a *visual mental state*. If this is the reading McGraw intends, his claim seems correct yet unsurprising: Certainly, while seeing a wall presupposes that there is a wall, it is not the same as a wall. The former is a mental event or state of the subject, the latter an (distinct) object in the world. Direct realists do not deny that there is a difference here.

The problem one might raise for a materialist with regard to the phenomenal qualities of perceptual states is the traditional worry of how phenomenal properties can be reduced to material or physical properties of the subject, such as functional properties or neural properties. One response to this problem that is available to direct realists with materialist commitments is to deny that there are any phenomenal properties of experience. This has been argued by Tye (2000) by appeal to the argument from transparency, for instance. (The argument says that there is no introspective evidence of qualia as intrinsic features of experience: When I try to focus on the phenomenal properties involved in experience, I inexorably end up with what experience presents as features of objects out there.) Crudely put, Tye's point is that the phenomenal character of experience is not to be understood in terms of qualitative properties that the experience *itself* has, but has to be reduced to what it represents, its content.

On the other hand, the visual impression might be the direct *object* sensed by the subject, something along the lines of a sense datum. Taken this way, McGraw's claim comes down to the indirect realist position that we are confronted with things in the world only indirectly, by immediately being in touch with sense data, ideas, or the like. As far as I can tell, this is the claim he is making. Compare the following quote (p. 23): "Human subjects are aware of the colors and other attributes that belong to physical objects as physical only by starting with phenomenal colors and attributes." According to McGraw, this is an undeniable fact about perceptual experience. But this is exactly what direct realism is committed to denying. On this view, what we are directly aware of in perception are features of the worldly things we perceive themselves. There *are no* impressions within in the perceiver that mediate her perception of her surroundings. In light of this, there is no need to worry about whether they, by contrast with worldly objects, stop existing when the subject looks away. If McGraw wants to argue otherwise, he needs to provide reasons why we should introduce such entities as impressions into our ontology in the first place.

But is there not still a problem for the direct realist? She says that the phenomenal character of perceptual experience is due to its object or content. (The exact claim varies, for instance, between intentionalist versions of direct realism such as Tye's and naïve realist versions such as Mike Martin's, 1997.) But, as McGraw argues, the features of physical things that we perceive are often categorically different from how these things strike us. For example, temperature is a statistical property and color is a complicated reflectance property, even though the warmth I feel or the shade of red that I see appears to be simple features of things around me (p. 4). While it would take me too far afield to elaborate on direct realist responses to this problem, let me point out that they can insist that we perceive complicated dispositional or statistical properties by perceiving their concrete manifestations. These manifestations are concrete properties instantiated by the perceived objects, so it is not surprising that they appear to be simple, intrinsic properties. Further, direct realists do not have to claim that our perceptual experiences give us full and transparent disclosure of the things they represent, including their physical structure or statistical properties.

A different response available to direct realists is to endorse a nonreductive materialism. John McDowell (1994), for instance, seems to be open to this view, which appeals to different, equally correct levels of description and explanation of reality. The undeniable directness of our perceptual engagement with the world is captured at the *personal* level of explanation. This does not conflict with the correctness of explanations at *subpersonal* levels of explanation, all the way down to the quantum level that describes and explains the world by appeal not to midsized objects but to atoms or the like.

What about the fact that the *phenomenal character* of seeing a wall vanishes once the subject looks away from the wall, whereas the wall, including its perceptible features, continues to exist? Does this not show that the phenomenal character of the subject's visual experience cannot arise from the wall and its properties? Direct realists can reply that the wall's visible features give rise to the phenomenal character of an experience of looking at the wall only when there is such an experience. But even when the subject looks away, the wall has these features that are available for her to perceive. It is in virtue of presenting her with these features that *this* is exactly what it is like for her to undergo the visual experience of the wall.

Toward the end of his contribution, McGraw himself appears to endorse a version of direct realism. He claims—quite plausibly—that the processes going on in the perceptual system are not something that obstructs the perceiver's contact with her surroundings. He also accepts the argument from transparency. I am not sure how to square these statements with his claim, quoted above, that we become aware of things in the world and their properties only via our contact with the phenomenal qualities of intramental impressions. Let me end my comment by suggesting that he should give up on this latter claim in favor of an all-out direct realist picture of perception.

PIERRE LE MORVAN'S COMMENTS ON BOB FRENCH'S "A DEFENSE OF REPRESENTATIONAL REALISM"

I enjoyed reading your paper. There has been such a swing back to direct realism in recent decades in the philosophy of perception that it's intellectually healthy to see someone vigorously defending representational (or indirect) realism as you did. As you might expect though, I am not convinced. Here are some comments that I hope you find helpful.

1. At numerous points in the paper, the position with which you contrast yours is what you call "naïve realism." In doing so, you seem (like many others in the literature) to be treating naïve realism as the only form of direct realism. To me, however, this is a mistake, for reasons I give in my own contribution. For instance, on p. 1, you write: "What I hold is responsible for the alleged directedness (reference) to the distal object under this account is just the mistaken assumption that this object is, in fact, immediately presented." You then give examples of illusions that tell against naïve realism and seem to suppose that they also tell against direct realism more broadly. However, a form of direct realism such as the Theory of Appearing is perfectly compatible with illusions and draws a distinction (that you do not) between causal and cognitive directness: just because something is not causally direct, it does not follow that it is not cognitively direct. In seeing a distal object, our seeing is causally indirect (as it involves a series of intermediate causal events including the passage of light rays), but it does not follow that the cognitively direct object (namely, what are aware of, what is presented to us) is something other than the distal object unless we assume indirect realism.

2. On p. 1 (second paragraph), you claim that "unlike the case with indirect realism where there is readily available physical explanation for these linkages (the passage of light rays between the distal objects and our eyes), it is incredibly unclear to me as to how any of these proposed mechanisms is to be instantiated." Note, however, that direct realists (at least philosophical ones) do not deny that the passage of light rays between the distal objects and our eyes is causally necessary for visual perception; what they deny is that it is conceptually or logically necessary therefor.

3. In discussing perceptual regress arguments, you argue on p. 6 (and elsewhere, e.g., p. 11) that "the ordinary language of perception is theory-laden, implicitly assuming the truth of naïve realism." I myself think this ordinary language is pretheoretical, but let us assume for the sake of argument that it is theory-laden. One advantage (ceteris paribus) of direct realism over indirect realism is that it does not call for the kind of reconstruction of our ordinary language that does your indirect realism, and it does not need to posit the kind of ambiguity of perceptual language you mention on p. 10.

4. If as you claim on p. 6 "the distinction between the 'senser' and the 'sensed' breaks down here; i.e., what is 'sensed' is held to just be a part of the conscious mind of the 'senser'" it seems to me that we are on the road to some form of idealism or phenomenalism. For as many (as Berkeley, Hegel, and many others) have pointed out, if the direct object of awareness is part of the conscious mind of the "senser," this fuels skepticism about there being mind-independent objects at all. Part the motivation for the return to direct realism over the past several decades is precisely this realization.

5. You argue (p. 37) that on the phenomenal reconstruction you propose, "if a regress is to be avoided here in the 'phenomenal' reconstruction of ordinary perceptual language, the perceptual verbs cannot be transitive. For example, using the 'phenomenal' reconstruction, an active voice equivalent to the passive voice 'redness is sensed (or apprehended) in a particular location in my phenomenal perceptual field' could be given here, whereby no distinction would be made between the portion of the senser's phenomenal field in which at a particular time (using the language of phenomenology) the object is 'constituted,' and what is 'sensed' or 'apprehended' at that time." If so, your view seems to amount to a form of adverbialism, which too denies the transitivity of perceptual verbs. This issue is worth clarifying.

MICHAEL HUEMER'S COMMENTS ON STEVEN LEHAR: THE "IRREFUTABLE" EVIDENCE FOR INDIRECT REALISM

1. THE ISSUE OF DIRECT AND INDIRECT REALISM

Steven Lehar defends a theory of perception that, he concedes, seems incredible on its face.[1] Yet he holds that the view must be accepted in the end because "in science, irrefutable evidence triumphs over incredibility."

I disagree that Lehar has presented irrefutable evidence for indirect realism or against direct realism. I think in fact that no evidence against direct realism has been given—not because the evidence Lehar cites is not true, but because it simply is not evidence *against direct realism*. In other words, Lehar's arguments are logically invalid; his conclusions do not follow from his premises.

---

[1] Lehar, S. The Epistemology of Visual Experience, this volume (Chapter 6).

To begin with, let us understand what direct and indirect realism are. In Lehar's formulation, *direct realism* holds "that the world we see around us is the world itself"; *indirect realism*, by contrast, holds "that the world we see around us is not the real world itself, but merely a perceptual replica of that world in an internal representation." (There are other ways of formulating the issue, but I propose for now to accept Lehar's formulation.[2]) So in what follows, the question to keep in mind is whether any of the evidence to be discussed supports the claim that the world we see is not the real (external, physical) world but merely an internal replica of the world.

2. THE CAUSAL ARGUMENT

Lehar's first argument against direct realism is very quick. Direct realism, he says, "is incredible because it suggests that we can have experience out beyond the sensory surface, in violation of everything we know about the causal chain of vision." By "everything we know about the causal chain of vision," I shall assume that Lehar is referring chiefly to the fact that certain electrochemical processes in the brain are causally necessary for vision or for perception in general. The argument against direct realism, then, seems to be something like this:

1. If direct realism is true, then our sensory experiences are spatially located outside our bodies.
2. Electrochemical processes in the brain are causally necessary for sensory experiences.
3. If processes in the brain are causally necessary for sensory experiences, then sensory experiences are located in our brains.
4. Therefore, direct realism is false.

Here, premise 1 is certainly false, so the remaining steps are immaterial. Direct realism does not hold that experiences are outside our bodies (which would indeed be a ridiculous view!). As Lehar originally stated the view, direct realism just holds that we perceive the real world. The claim that we perceive the real world does not imply anything about the spatial location of our experiences, if indeed experiences have spatial locations at all.

---

[2] Elsewhere, I have formulated the issue in terms of whether we have direct awareness of external phenomena, where direct awareness is awareness that is not based on awareness of anything else; see my 2001, Ch. IV. Points similar to those I make below in the text can be made also for this more sophisticated formulation of the issue.

Perhaps Lehar intended the argument to be something more like this:

The Perception Argument

P1. For me to perceive (e.g.,) a table, it is causally necessary that certain electrochemical processes occur in my brain.

P2. Therefore, I cannot perceive an external, physical table; I can only perceive a replica of a table in my head.

P1 is true. But P2 neither follows from P1 nor provides any evidence for P2. Compare the following argument for a view we might dub "automotive indirect realism":

The Car Argument

C1. For me to drive a car, it is causally necessary that certain electrochemical processes occur in my muscles.

C2. Therefore, I cannot drive an external, physical car. I can only drive a replica of a car in my muscles.

The Car Argument is invalid. C1 is true, but C2 obviously does not follow and is not true. Since the Perception Argument and the Car Argument have the same logical form, either both are valid or both are invalid. So both are invalid.

Part of the process of normal perception involves events in the brain. That is well known and disputed by no one. But the fact that perception involves events in the brain does not mean that *what we perceive* is something in our brains. What we perceive (the *objects* of our perception) is not to be confused either with the process of perceiving or with the causal conditions of our perceiving.

Similarly, the process of driving a car involves events in our muscles, but this does not mean that *what* one drives is something in one's muscles.[3]

3. DREAMS, HALLUCINATIONS, AND ILLUSIONS

Lehar's second argument also goes by quickly: "The phenomena of dreams and hallucinations are problematic for Direct [Realism] because they demonstrate the capacity of the brain to construct complete virtual worlds, a capacity which must surely be employed also in normal spatial perception, as revealed by many visual illusions."

I do not think dreams and hallucinations are problematic for direct realism. Granted, when one dreams or hallucinates, one does not perceive the real world. This does not entail that in normal perception, one does not perceive the real world. It does not even *provide evidence* that in normal perception, one does not perceive the real world. That is because we know why dreams

---

[3] For further discussion, see my 2001, pp. 79–85, 135.

and hallucinations do not count as perceptions of real objects, and we know that this reason does not apply to normal perception. The reason dreams and hallucinations do not count as perceptions of real objects is that, when one dreams or hallucinates, one's experience is not caused by a real object of the sort that appears to be present. This is just a conceptual point. But normal perceptions *are* caused by real objects of the sort that appear to be present.

Here is an analogy. For someone to count as *knowing* A (where A is any proposition), A has to be true. For instance, you cannot know that it's raining unless it is in fact raining. False beliefs do not count as knowledge. But this neither implies nor provides any evidence for the claim that *true* beliefs do not count as knowledge. The brain's capacity for forming false beliefs does not show that no belief is knowledge. Similarly, the brain's capacity for having experiences that do not correspond to reality does not show that no experience is a perception of reality.

What about the case of visual illusions? Here is a favorite example among skeptics: if you look at a straight stick that is half submerged in water, the stick will often appear bent. Does this show that direct realism is false?

Again, remember what the issue was: do we perceive real, physical objects, or do we perceive replicas of objects in our heads? The bent stick illusion does not show that you perceive a copy of the stick in your head. Rather, you see the stick (the real, physical stick, for that is the only sticklike thing there is), which *looks* bent but *is* straight. The fact that it looks bent does not mean that it is a stick rèplica in your head.[4]

4. THE GEOMETRICAL ARGUMENT

I turn to Lehar's main original contribution. This is the argument that visual space (the space in which the things we see appear) is non-Euclidean, whereas real, physical space is Euclidean (or close enough for our purposes). Therefore, says Lehar, the space in which the objects we see appear is not physical space. Therefore, these objects themselves are not the real, physical objects. Here is Lehar:

> [P]henomenal perspective embodies [a] contradiction in terms, with parallel lines meeting at two points while passing to either side of the percipient, and while being perceived to be straight and parallel and equidistant throughout their length. This absurd contradiction is clearly not a property of the physical world, which is measurably Euclidean at least at the familiar scale of our everyday environment. Therefore, that curvature must be a property of perceived space…

[4] For further discussion of illusion and hallucination, see my 2001, pp. 124–129.

Here, the argument seems to be that visual space has contradictory properties; therefore, it cannot be identical with physical space. But if the premise is true, then the proper conclusion would not be that visual space is in your head, or in your mind, rather than being in the outside world. The proper conclusion would be that visual space does not exist. *Nothing* can have contradictory properties, wherever it may be. Locating an object in a person's head does not enable that object to defy the laws of logic.

(By the way, this is not to be confused with the question of whether a person can have contradictory beliefs or other mental states. A person may be able to believe contradictory propositions, but a person cannot have a belief that itself *has contradictory properties*—for instance, being both a belief and not a belief. The same is true of any mental state, brain state, or anything else.)

But how should we describe visual experience? When one looks at a pair of train tracks that recede very far into the distance, do they appear parallel or not? And do they appear to meet in the distance or not?

The tracks only *sort of* appear to meet in the distance. That is, one's visual experience is *similar to* (but not *indistinguishable from*) the visual experience one has when one looks at, say, a painting of train tracks, in which the lines on the canvas would actually meet.

What is actually true is neither that the train tracks definitely *appear to meet* nor that they *appear not to meet*; rather, as the tracks get farther away, it becomes increasingly difficult to tell, by direct visual inspection (without moving), whether they continue to be parallel. If the tracks are sufficiently long, one simply *cannot tell* whether they meet at some point or not. (Imagine a trick set of train tracks, where the tracks actually get a millimeter closer together with every 100 m, and eventually meet far away. This pair of tracks might be visually indistinguishable from a normal pair in which the tracks are parallel.)

Compare another interesting phenomenon, that of "color constancy." Try looking at a red apple in a well-lit room, then looking at the same apple outside at night. Does the apple appear the same color? *In one sense*, the apple continues to look red when outside at night. If someone asked you, outside at night, to visually determine the apple's color, you would say, "It is red." But in another sense, everything looks a dark, bluish gray.

Now, imagine someone saying: "The apple you see is both red and bluish gray at the same time. But no physical object can have such contradictory properties. So you must be seeing a nonphysical object." That is crazy. *No* object can have contradictory properties, so nothing is both red and bluish gray at the same time—it does not matter whether it be physical or mental.

A better description is that the apple *sort of* looks red and *sort of* looks bluish gray. This shows that visual experience can have different levels of content coexisting. It does not show that there is some apple-like object that *is red* and at the same time *is bluish gray*.

Similarly, train tracks receding in the distance sort of appear to get closer together and sort of appear parallel. But this does not show that there is some pair of objects with contradictory properties, whether in your head or elsewhere.

Note, incidentally, that if Lehar's geometrical argument were correct, it would commit him to mind–body dualism. His argument turns on the premise that objects in visual space have properties that no physical object has. That entails that there are nonphysical objects, so dualism is true. I myself have no objection to dualism, but Lehar seems to want to avoid dualism.

5. WHAT KIND OF THEORY IS DIRECT REALISM?

Indirect realists often think that direct realism is a silly empirical error, founded on overlooking extremely widespread and well-known empirical facts (indeed, facts which have in essence been known for hundreds or thousands of years). Hence, Steven Lehar appeals to "irrefutable evidence."

By contrast, I do not think indirect realism is an empirical oversight. I think it is a *confusion*. I think indirect realism results from such conceptual mistakes as: confusing an *object* of perception with the *process* of perceiving, confusing the way objects *appear* with the way they *are*, confusing causal indirectness with epistemological indirectness, and especially confusing a representation with that which is represented. The idea that we can only perceive perceptions is like the idea that we can only discuss words, that we can only think about thoughts, or that we can only depict depictions. The truth or falsity of these ideas is not a scientific issue, and there are no experiments that could be done to resolve it.

Lehar writes that "in the end this is a paradigm debate over whether vision is truly magical and beyond scientific explanation." No, it is not. The question is not whether perception is magical. The question is whether any of the well-known facts about perception—that we have sensory experiences, that we sometimes experience illusions, that there are internal causal preconditions on perception—show that we do not really perceive physical objects. My answer is that, as a conceptual matter, they simply do not show anything of the kind.

REFERENCES

Austin, J.L., 1962. Sense and Sensibilia. Clarendon Press, Oxford.
Berkeley, G., 2008. The principles of human knowledge. In: Clarke, D. (Ed.), George Berkeley, Philosophical Writings. Cambridge University Press, Cambridge.
Brewer, B., 2008. How to account for illusion. In: Haddock, A., Macpherson, F. (Eds.), Disjunctivism: Perception, Action, Knowledge. Oxford University Press, Oxford, pp. 168–180.
Huemer, M., 2001. Skepticism and the Veil of Perception. Rowman & Littlefield, Lanham, MD.
Martin, M.G.F., 1997. The reality of appearances. In: Sainsbury, M. (Ed.), Thought and Ontology. FrancoAngeli, Milan, pp. 81–106.
Martin, M., 2009. The reality of experiences. In: Byrne, A., Logue, H. (Eds.), Disjunctivism: Contemporary Readings. MIT Press, Cambridge, MA, pp. 91–116.
McDowell, J., 1994. Mind and World. Harvard University Press, Cambridge, MA.
Ryle, G., 1949. The Concept of Mind. Hutchinson's University Library, London.
Tye, M., 1995. Ten Problems of Consciousness. MIT Press, Cambridge, MA.
Tye, M., 2000. Consciousness, Color, and Content. MIT Press, Cambridge, MA.

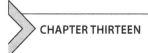

Critiques of Papers by Direct Realists by Indirect Realists

Robert French
Adjunct Instructor, Philosophy, Oakland Community College, Waterford Township, MI, United States

ROBERT FRENCH'S COMMENTS ON MICHAEL HUEMER

In his paper Michael Huemer presents a defense of an epistemological version of Direct Realism. Some epistemological versions may even be compatible with at least metaphysical versions of Indirect Realism. However, as Eva Schmidt argues in her selection (in the context of discussing disjunctivism) this is slippery. In particular, Huemer's version clearly is not compatible with Indirect Realism, as even he concedes. Thus, I confine my remarks to Huemer's version as given and even within these confines the remarks are incomplete in that they do not touch on everything, which Huemer covers.

Huemer claims that experiences are external world propositions and thus makes them conceptual. In particular he construes experiences in terms of a special type of propositional attitude. Instead I hold that they are clearly spatial events occurring in a private phenomenal space. This may be hidden in Huemer's definition of "phenomenal conservatism" where Huemer uses "seems" to refer to a propositional attitude. "Seems" is a notoriously ambiguous term, which Dennett (1991, p. 131), for example, fails to distinguish in an equivocation between phenomenal and propositional senses. I believe that Huemer takes advantage of the same ambiguity since I hold that phenomenal seemings are spatial and not propositional.

In Chapter 7, Sections 2.2 and 2.3, illustrations are given of two illusions—the Müller-Lyer illusion and the duck-rabbit ambiguous picture; also used by Wittgenstein (1953, par. II, sec. xi). Huemer claims that the differences just involve matters of interpretation—external world propositions. In contrast, I hold that the illusions are constructed in phenomenal visual space with different geometric structures due to the ambiguities in depth cues; e.g., in the Müller-Lyer illusion the line, which is perceived as being longer, has perspectival depth cues for being more distant than its surround

Direct versus Indirect Realism
ISBN 978-0-12-812141-2
https://doi.org/10.1016/B978-0-12-812141-2.00013-1

© 2018 Elsevier Inc.
All rights reserved.

and thus due to the tendency toward size constancy is reconstructed longer in phenomenal visual space.

With respect to Reid, in Huemer's quote from Section 4.1 of his *Inquiry into the Human Mind*, (1764/1970) Reid explicitly states that he is referring to perception not sensation and distinguishes between the two. In particular, Reid holds that perception is an indirect process whereby sensations (which are in the conscious mind) serve as natural signs for distal physical objects. He then tries to escape skepticism by, in a move somewhat reminiscent of Berkeley, invoking God—the artist in the passage.

Also, in the *Inquiry*, Reid postulates a spherical geometry for vision (discussed in his section on the "geometry of visibles"). It is noteworthy that the discussion of a spherical geometry for vision is not also included in Reid's (1785/1969) *Essays on the Intellectual Powers of Man* where he explicitly does espouse a version of Direct Realism, at least for color. Admittedly there are issues concerning how to interpret Reid (since he claims throughout his works to be avoiding the skeptical implications of empiricism) and since in his inquiry he does define "visibles" as solid angles subtended by retinal images.

Reid also claims both that visual appearances and visible figures lack thickness, even though he analyzes the former as sensations and the latter as visibles. To my mind that shows that he often does not clearly distinguish between the two. He even states that the only reason he does not hold that visibles are sensations is that using David Hume's language impressions (waking sensations) and ideas (nonwaking experiences) are nonspatial. This is an assumption, which definitely can be questioned. In any event the goal here should be a search for what is actually going on, not just an exegesis of Reid.

In Section 4.4 in the discussion of acquaintance it should be emphasized that Russell (1912) uses William James's (1890, Ch. 8) phrase "knowledge by acquaintance" to refer to knowledge of sense data. Later in his career Russell (1948) also uses the phrase to refer to knowledge of events in a private phenomenal space. He never uses it for knowledge claims about our physical environment, which he calls knowledge by description. Even though Huemer does not claim that noninferential justification requires acquaintance but instead only appearances, if appearances are direct and not indirect perceptions, it is not clear to me how to distinguish between the two.

Except for cases of compelling illusions such as the Ames rooms or so-called 3D movies I concede that for almost all practical situations the attitude of Naïve Realism (taking our experiences of distal objects for at least the front surfaces of those objects) works fine and thus need not be repudiated for purposes of practical life. I think that Huemer is right that in these sorts of circumstances the ordinary person does not consciously make an inference to the existence of a distal object of perception. However, I also hold though that this is only because the ordinary person mistakenly takes the phenomenal appearance for the front surface of that distal object. I believe that these last comments are important since they both explain why the attitude of Naïve Realism works as well as it does and also why this does not establish that it is fundamental.

I agree with Huemer's claim that the epistemology for external world propositions is more straightforward on a Direct Realist account of perception since it holds that we possess an immediate appearance of these objects. However, it is possible for an Indirect Realist to rationally reconstruct senses of "knowledge" in nonillusory contexts that work for at least most practical purposes. None of these senses involve claims to certainty and thus do not completely capture the ordinary language meaning of "knowledge." These rational reconstructions include Goldman's (1979) reliability account and various pragmatic accounts (such as those given by various American pragmatists) that at least work for most commonly encountered environments; e.g., those consisting of what Austin (1962, p. 8) calls "moderate-sized specimens of dry goods." When encountering these sorts of situations it is true that we usually get away with taking the conscious visual experience for the front surface of the distal physical object. Also, since these senses lack certainty various moves are necessary to get around Gettier-like (1963) counterexamples, although I will not develop this point further.

Finally, I wish to emphasize that none of the foregoing is truly fundamental with respect to knowledge of the physical world. To understand what is actually going on in one's physical environment one needs to use the methods of the physical science i.e., the hypothetical deductive method where certainty is never attained. Noteworthily the best resulting model postulated by physics (look at quantum physics, for example) is incredibly different from the way that world is reconstructed in perception.

ROBERT FRENCH'S COMMENTS ON WILLIAM FISH

In his paper William Fish develops an interesting (and possibly significant) variant on a disjunctive theory of perception, giving a phenomenal version of it. Within the context of Direct Realism Fish also presents an interesting discussion of the concept of "screening off" whereby a common property (e.g., being phenomenal) inherits the explanatory potential of a special property (e.g., being a veridical percept). It should be emphasized off the bat that Fish's version of disjunctivism is significantly different from epistemological and metaphysical versions of disjunctivism and can also be seen as a retreat from those positions, due to mentioned difficulties with them. Also, it should be pointed out at the onset that Fish's theory differs from traditional versions of Naïve Realism to the extent that theory is held to be identical with the theory of perception of common sense. This is because common sense does not take the front surfaces of objects to be seen as being phenomenal, but instead holds that their format of existence is nonmental. I only comment on portions of Fish's paper, almost exclusively from Part II where he develops his positive theory.

Fish's theory appears to have at least some affinities with the neutral monism of James (1904) and later Russell (1921). Unlike James's and Russell's versions of neutral monism though, Fish's theory is also disjunctive in character in that he holds that veridical and nonveridical perception lack common content since they differ in phenomenal character. However, Fish does not specify how these respective contents differ in phenomenal character. Also, Fish cannot make the standard move that these contents are at least numerically distinct inasmuch as he does not hold the causal theory of perception in at least its standard form whereby even veridical percepts are held to be at least numerically distinct from their distal physical objects. It should be emphasized as well that during his career Russell (1921, 1927, 1948) progressively moved away from neutral monism, as he became better aware of how incredibly different the microscopic world of quantum physics is from our perception of distal objects. In his later works Russell clearly endorses a causal theory of perception where he distinguishes between mental events in phenomenal space and phenomenal time and nonmental events in physical space and physical time.

I believe that there is nothing neutral about the position of neutral monism. While some who agree with me on this claim believe that the so-called "neutral elements" are actually physical and not mental, I hold that the reverse is clearly the case. In particular, I hold that these elements are clearly mental both since the physical realm, at least as described by modern quantum physics, is so different from our experiences of it and since the concept of the "phenomenal" is by definition a sensual, and hence a mental, concept. I believe that this may be missed by Naïve Realists since I hold that they misidentify veridical and many illusory experiences for physical front surfaces. In contrast, I hold that the actual physical front surfaces transcend (in the sense of lying beyond) these phenomena. Apropos to this point when Fish gives the example of Pauline veridically sensing the redness of an apple, it would help to distinguish between phenomenal and physical senses of color. They are very different; a fact that is hidden by ordinary language since it does not make the distinction.

Fish denies that there is any common content between cases of veridical perception and cases of hallucination and in the reference given, goes so far as to claim that hallucinations lack phenomenal content, although holding that they do possess cognitive features of "anomalous beliefs." I find these claims to be implausible. Consider cases of after-images, (which are cases of hallucination if these are defined as nonveridical experiences since they are not caused by distal objects) which possess complementary phenomenal colors to the veridical percepts. These do not just involve "anomalous beliefs," but rather possess a spatial structure. Also, there is no entirely sharp distinction between cases of hallucination and cases of illusion. Consider the blind spot. In spite of there being no photoreceptors at the site where the optic nerve exits the retina there is no corresponding gap in phenomenal visual experience. Instead, an interpolation from surrounding photoreceptors is used to "fill in" the phenomenal color. Something similar occurs with the case of the Krauskopf (1963) effect discussed by Ernest Kent in his contribution to this volume. Numerous examples from fields such as ventriloquism and magic shows can also be cited where phenomenal reconstructions are very different from their distal physical objects.

Other points include Fish's use of Putnam's term "cognition powers" to serve as the function by means of which a "veil of perception" or interface reaches out to a distal object rather than experiential object. In my opinion it would be better to speak of "experiencing" these objects inasmuch as the use of "cognitive powers" would appear to be compatible with the use of indirect means. Even if cognition in this context is construed as a case of "knowledge by acquaintance," as that term, for example, is developed by both James and Russell, as Russell clearly points out such a construal does not constitute knowledge of physical objects but rather mental sense data.

Like Russell and Locke I wish to defend the existence of phenomenal interfaces in perception. The one objection, which Fish raises here, is an epistemic one concerning how we can gain cognitive access to the distal objects. All that I wish to say is that we must settle for a sense of cognition here that is less than that of certainty, as outlined in my other replies. Admittedly there are also issues, which can be raised concerning the ontological status of such interfaces, such as whether or not they are reducible to brain states as with certain versions of identity theories and dual aspect theories, which hold that there are neural correlates of consciousness. However, since anything like an adequate discussion would take at least another full-length book, I will not deal with these issues here.

⟩⟩ ROBERT FRENCH'S COMMENTS ON EVA SCHMIDT

In her paper Eva Schmidt presents a compelling dilemma for knowledge-based or epistemological versions of disjunctive accounts of perception. In one horn of the dilemma the position collapses into a metaphysical version of Direct Realism, which appears to be the same as Naïve Realism holding that we possess immediate conscious awareness of at least aspects of distal objects of perception. The problems for such a position are well known. The other horn of the dilemma is what John McDowell (1982/2009) has termed a "highest common factor view," which refers to "what is available to experience in the deceptive and nondeceptive cases alike" and where there are "substantial mental commonalities" between cases of hallucinations and cases of veridical perception. As far as I can see the highest common factor view, in effect, is an Indirect Realist position. If this is true then in spite of surface appearances Schmidt's paper does not just concern an internal debate among Direct Realist positions. Instead she is arguing that the only possibly viable version of externalism or Direct Realism is the metaphysical version. If this position does not hold up, we are left with some version of Indirect Realism. Schmidt does not present any arguments against this position other than merely to state her preference for disjunctivism.

I am willing to grant that when confined to the topic of Direct Realist theories, what Schmidt argues for may have considerable merit. However, while I grant that if one assumes her assumptions, that the case for the metaphysical version of a disjunctive account of perception may be compelling I do not accept these assumptions. This is because I hold an Indirect Realist position. Another point is that, like many Direct Realists, Schmidt claims that the contents of perception are propositional when she states that they are facts. I take it that by 'facts' Schmidt is referring to true propositions, but if instead she is trying to refer to a nonlinguistic account, such as the one, which Fish (2009, pp. 53, 54) tries to give, this should be specified. For example, Schmidt uses the locution "sees that there is a red box" where the object is propositional. However, notice that this already involves a verbal interpretation of the object, which goes beyond the object per se. It is not obvious that this move also works if one instead speaks of "seeing the red box" since one can do this even if one lacks the concept of a box.

Even within the context of Direct Realist theories I have a major problem with the claim that the objects of perception are propositional. Objects of perception (even if they are directly perceived) would seem to be the features of the world described by the relevant propositions themselves, rather than being the propositions per se. I take these objects to be spatial states of affairs—whether construed as by Direct Realists in a public nonmental physical space, or as I take them to be, events in a private phenomenal space. These states of affairs make factual claims be true, but, if facts are construed as being conceptual, I do not think that these facts themselves are perceived; although we can speak of "perceiving that" some fact is the case.

It is true that in Chapter 10, footnote 2 Schmidt says that her arguments also goes through if you conceive of perception as being directed at objects. I take it that she is referring to distal physical objects here, or at least the front surfaces of them, in which case the position sounds a lot like traditional Naïve Realism, such as G.E. Moore's (1959) version. My basic disagreement then is that what I hold, using the attitude of common sense, we take as the distal front surface, I hold in fact consists of phenomenal colors in our private phenomenal spaces. The distal object still exists, but only as atoms reflecting various light rays, which causally connect me with the object. For most practical purposes (i.e., for practical knowledge, which the ancient Greeks called Φρόνησις), apart from some of the more compelling illusions, we get away with taking one for the other.

 ## ROBERT FRENCH'S COMMENTS ON PIERRE LE MORVAN

In his paper Pierre Le Morvan purports to distinguish among the different variants of perceptual realism—the position that perception-independent physical objects are what perceivers perceive. Le Morvan carefully distinguishes among a number of variants of Direct Realist theories of perception. Unfortunately I find what Le Morvan says concerning Indirect Realism not to be consistent and also quite sketchy. In his introduction Le Morvan contrasts Perceptual Realism with sense-data theories, many of which are paradigm cases of Indirect Realist theories of perception. However, in Section 3 Le Morvan claims that Indirect Realism is a version of Perceptual Realism. He says very little about Indirect Realism—citing only Descartes and Locke, while ignoring such 20th century figures as Bertrand Russell during the 1940s (Russell, 1940, 1948) and John Smythies (1994).

I agree that Direct Realism has many different variants and that it is important to identify, which variants are being either defended or critiqued.

However, Indirect Realism has at least as many variants and some of these variants (particularly epistemic ones) may even be compatible with some variants of Direct Realism. Versions can also be distinguished on such issues as to whether any mediate objects, which Indirect Realists postulate the existence of are characterized as being spatial or nonspatial (e.g., conceptual) and on whether these mediate objects are postulated to be brain states, functions of such states or something else.

One important issue, which should be raised, is that there is a danger that someone may shift among (or retreat from) different variants of Naïve Realism for the sole purpose of escaping refutations. For example, in his discussion of different versions of "local Naïve Realisms" Le Morvan distinguishes among temporal (perceive at the same time), chromatic (perceive as having the same color), formal (perceive as having the same shape or structure), and motional (perceive as having the same motion) versions along with other variants. Each of these variants is easily refutable by citing differences between the relevant perceptions and their distal objects with respect to each of these respective properties.

I wish also now to point out a danger with the process of shifting among these different variants of Naïve Realism. This danger is that it may make the position of Naïve Realism in general impossible to tie down to any set-specific content and thus also to be impossible to refute. This is never a healthy attitude in any field—Karl Popper (1972) terms it as "immunizing a theory against refutation." In fact there is also a thesis in the philosophy of science, the Quine–Duhem thesis (Quine, 1951; Duhem, 1906/1954), that any claim can be saved if one is willing to make enough other changes in one's system. Imre Lakatos (1970) has called this a "regressive research program," and I have at least some fear that what has been happening with the current plethora of mutually incompatible Direct Realist theories of perception may constitute such a program.

ROBERT FRENCH'S COMMENTS ON FRED ADAMS

Since most of the paper of Adams et al. is directed at my paper in this volume I will confine my comments to a response to what they say concerning that paper. Also, while I have major disagreements with what they assert about my position in more than one section of the paper I will focus my comments on just one issue, which I believe is the key one. This issue concerns the nature of the relationship between the veridical experiences of a perceiver and the distal objet perceived. Adams et al. claim that Indirect

Realists posit three-place relations here. This may be true of some Indirect Realist theories, but it is not true of mine. Instead, I, like Adams et al., hold that it is a two-place relation since I do not hold that there is an intervening object in between the experiences of the perceiver and the distal object perceived. I believe that our differences in fact lie elsewhere as I will now elaborate.

Adams et al. and I agree on the nature of the external relatum—the distal object of perception, which we agree possesses an independent existence apart from being perceived. However, we disagree both on the nature of the first relatum and on the nature of the linkage between the two. I will deal with these two topics separately.

With respect to the nature of the first relatum, I explicitly deny that the experience either represents an internal phenomenal state or represents itself. Therein lies the way of regresses, such as in talk of being aware of experiences (the awareness is the experience). Instead I hold that experiences per se are constituted by events in a private phenomenal space. This is a key consideration with respect to what Adams et al. assert with respect to my remarks concerning a phenomenal regress. It is not so much that reconstructing perceptual language solves the regress as that it created it in the first place by forcing a distinction between perceivers and what is perceived by using transitive verbs. This needs to be pointed out to resolve matters. I also deny that experiences are cognitive states at least if these are construed as anything possessing just a conceptual nature.

It is true that Adams et al. invoke qualitative properties of the experiences (which they term "qualia") and mental representations here, which they claim constitute information about the distal object. That this is a very different position from the older representational tradition may be hidden since Adams, following Dretske and Tye, have co-opted some of the language—in particular "representational," "phenomenal content," and "qualia"—from the representational tradition, which is much older dating back at least to Locke and Descartes and even to Plato with his allegory of the cave. I will make a few remarks on the story with "representational" first and will move on to "phenomenal content" and "qualia."

The use of "representational," is very old and was used to refer to a version of Indirect Realism whereby sense data were held to represent their distal objects both by resemblance and causal relationships. It was then co-opted by at least some Direct Realists to refer to their own position. For example, Edmond Wright, who was writing a paper "One Answer to the Accusation of Relativism" for this volume before his unfortunate death in

2016, points out (Wright, 2008, p. 2) that Tye (1995) calls his own version of Direct Realism a representational theory in spite of its previous usage to refer to theories in the sense-datum tradition.

I will treat the cases of phenomenal content and qualia together since I do not see a distinction between them. Following Dretske's 1995 analysis Adams et al. construe both "phenomenal content" and "qualia" in terms of representations of distal objects. Completely mechanical systems (thermostats for Adams, speedometers for Dretske) are even cited in this analysis. Dretske (1995, p. 22) even speaks of the "speed qualia" of the speedometer. It is true that Adams et al. are somewhat more circumspect, denying, for example, that thermostats per se possess phenomenal content. However, they do ascribe phenomenal content to a physical neural haptic system selectively firing with respect to a keypad. At least to me it is both not clear what the key features are for distinguishing between the two cases and why they would be key. The only point I wish to make concerning the usage of Dretske and Adams et al. is that this is emphatically not the way the term "qualia" is used in the phenomenology tradition.

With respect to the subject of linkages between veridical experiences and their distal objects, Adams et al. mention Dretske's concept of a primary representation. Something like this is required to create a unique "experience" or representation of a distal object. However, Dretske provides two incompatible analyses here; one, Dretske (1981, p. 160), in terms of information theory and one, Dretske (1981, p. 162), in terms of "proper qualities." Adams et al. use the latter definition when they speak of what is "best correlated." Aside from being incredibly vague on the issue of what variables are relevant for constituting the best correlations there are also problems with uniqueness. Even with Dretske's restriction that the correlated object possess nomic (lawlike even in counterfactual conditions) relations with their distal objects, there are obvious problematic cases such as cases of mirror images and seeing something on live (or even taped) television. Even our language is not consistent here since we speak of seeing someone in a mirror or on television but may also speak of seeing the mirror surface or the television screen. We even speak of seeing the distal object in cases of using optical instruments containing mirrors as with some binoculars or reflecting telescopes.

An added issue is how veridical perceptual experiences "reach out to" their distal objects. Adams et al. and I agree that this involves causal chains but disagree on how. While their account, as given, is quite sketchy, Adams et al. hold that we are in direct contact with distal objects by means of a primary representation of that object by information concerning it. I take it that this is the alternative version of Direct Realism that is mentioned in the paper as differing from Naïve Realism. An obvious problem for this position is that, as I point out in my paper, while the information may be in common, this at most would establish a qualitative identity in at least some respects and does not constitute numerical identity. I completely fail to see how such a representation could constitute directly coming into contact with the distal object.

In contrast to the version of Direct Realism of Adams et al., I hold that neural events in the brain—neural correlates of consciousness—produce a reconstruction of certain features of the distal object in a private phenomenal space. I then hold that in ordinary life, using the common sense attitude of Naïve Realism, we then take (or better mistake) the private phenomenal spatial experience for the distal object. As I point out in my paper this works for most, but not all (e.g., cases of compelling illusions), practical purposes.

A final point is that in their discussion of illusions Adams et al. state that they do not believe that "phenomenal objects exist." The phrase "phenomenal object" is radically ambiguous, but I think that they are referring to sense data or, in my language, events in a private phenomenal space then. If this is the case then I suspect that Adams et al. have mistaken events in private phenomenal space for what they take to be the physical objects, which they claim we are in contact with when it is alleged that we experience the world. It should be further emphasized that with illusions such as the Müller-Lyer illusion or those associated with random-dot stereograms it is the very spatial structure of phenomenal visual space, which is changed and not just an issue of conceptual. In effect Adams et al. give an adverbial account of illusions whereby visual cues distort the appearance of the actual objects. They claim that there are no phenomenal perceptual objects here but only, I take it, the distorted aspects of the distal object. Such an account is going to have to go into great convolutions to account for the effects of 3D movies. It is much more straightforward to say that these effects are due to a reconstruction from binocular depth cues.

DAVID MCGRAW'S COMMENTS ON EVA SCHMIDT, "DILEMMA FOR EPISTEMOLOGICAL DISJUNCTIVISM"

On the whole, the paper seems good enough, but two points stand out in my mind.

To take the lesser point first, there is the complaint over the proposal of object-dependent Fregean propositions (Chapter 10, page 150, footnote 2). This is said to overintellectualize what happens with perceptual experience.

Well, maybe and maybe not. True, that is not generally what happens with most people, but this fact may be more of a challenge to the people. Of course, the objection seems right about this particular proposal, but the complaint about over intellectualizing is much more questionable. The truth could turn out to be, experience based on perceiving through the senses is of fairly low epistemic value apart from some rather strict and well-developed mental discipline. I am not the first to raise this concern.

Going on to the second and more serious point, there is what is said at the end against the answer of hallucination as merely wayward perception (Chapter 10, pp. 156 and 157). This objection fails. When Louis the lifeguard sees a child drowning, he does *not* know that the child is drowning simply because she is drowning. If that were all it took, the whole of concrete reality would be open to him. But in fact, much of concrete reality is opaque to him and hidden from him. No, but instead, he knows the child is drowning because his own functioning has made him aware of this fact. True, he observes the fact only because it is there to be observed. In that sense, and in that sense only, yes, he is aware of the fact because there is the fact. However, this point is not contrary to the thesis that veridical observation is the starting point, and hallucination is merely wayward perception.

1. DAVID MCGRAW'S COMMENTS ON WILLIAM FISH

What Professor Fish says seems right. What he says about direct access, and about the need to say the import of hallucinations is parasitic on that of veridical experiences, looks to be correct. So far, so good. However, what he says does not really seem to have any bearing either on the question of materialism or on that of Naïve Realism as traditionally understood.

The point of saying "as traditionally understood" is that he gives his own definition of Naïve Realism. Quite clearly, his definition is too weak to capture what is at stake in the traditional debates. To be sure, the claim that the conscious character of the experience someone has on seeing an object could not have been the same in the absence of the object is certainly part of what is involved in traditional Naïve Realism. But this claim does not reach the usual question of whether this conscious character is, so to speak, a direct transcription or reflection of the object's character.

This point can be brought out clearly with the old inverted spectrum problem. Given that Wendy experiences phenomenal red where Beatrice experiences phenomenal violet, and vice versa, what then? Professor Fish's version of Naïve Realism could very well apply to, or be true of, both ladies. Wendy and Beatrice might each be able to say truly, "The conscious character of my experience would not be the same if the real object in the material world were not there." But the traditional version cannot possibly be true of both. The real color of the real light in the material world that reaches someone's eye cannot directly match both red and violet, or both yellow and blue, and so on. To be sure, both ladies may be experiencing veridically, in the sense that each lady's experience can be appropriately mapped into the material world. But that is not the same thing.

2. DAVID MCGRAW'S COMMENTS ON MICHAEL HUEMER

Huemer disclaims concern here with the nature and function of conscious experience as such. What he says seems to be compatible with either the affirmation or denial of traditional Naïve Realism and also with either the affirmation or denial of materialism. Nothing he says lends any support to the claim that these two could be combined. That being so, my concerns for the anthology do not reach what he says in this essay.

As for what he is concerned with, at least some version of it is most likely true. What he says is very much along the line that conscious experience is diaphanous or transparent, which I take over from Moore (and from Aristotle long before that). Experiences point *to objects* and not to themselves as mental events. Thus, to have conscious experience is already to have some sort of presumptive evidence for the presence and function of real objects behind the experience. What he says about appearance would seem to be another version of this basic idea.

"But how do you know you are not a brain in a vat in a laboratory, with electrodes attached, and so on?" I know it in the same way I know in the first place that there are such things as brains, vats, laboratories, and electrodes. This answer is much closer to what Huemer develops than to the theories he criticizes. This kind of skeptic takes over part of the framework developed out of experience and uses it to call the whole framework into question. He is not really entitled to do this. In taking over the part of the framework he uses, the skeptic has already committed himself to a whole lot of the apparatus of classical realism.

Then again, this skeptical usage would be legitimate if the skeptic could show that the part he uses breaks down on its own terms or goes against other essential points of classical realism. To say sensory experience must be vindicated by reason is right insofar as the question is whether classical realism leads into irresolvable paradoxes. But to show that this question is at stake would require going far beyond the brain in a vat challenge. Unless and until it is shown, Huemer's answer would seem to be right.

The great challenge comes with the claim that experience is diaphanous or transparent, to which he seems committed. To make this work, it seems Huemer must accept either Naïve Realism or some (suitably reconstructed) version of the old Aristotelian theory. But the essay here leaves it open which way he should go. Nothing here compels him to come down on one side or the other of that question. As for what the right answer is, that is a debate for another day.

ERNEST W. KENT'S COMMENTS ON MICHAEL HUEMER: COMMENT ON "THE VIRTUES OF DIRECT REALISM" BY MICHAEL HUEMER

Dr. Huemer asserts that Direct Realism would provide noninferential evidence for the external, physical world from perception, while Indirect Realism provides only inferential evidence. He presents reasons why he prefers the former.

He allows that "inferential justification" may include unconscious or implicit inference. There is a vast literature on mechanisms of unconscious determinants of perceptual experience, which include perceptual learning, imprinting, and evolutionary factors among others, and these would certainly then fall under the heading of "unconscious" or "implicit" inference. I perceive my environment in certain ways because it has been useful to my evolutionary forebears to do so, or because I have been exposed to certain pairings of sensations with events at developmentally critical periods that have modified my perceptions to attune my behavior to the particular idiosyncrasies of stimuli in my environment, or because my perceptual processes have adapted as a result of repeatedly experienced results of acting on perceptual information. I see what appears to be an obstacle at a certain distance and it is confirmed when I bump my nose on it, and my distance perception is thereby refined. It would seem then that unless the perceptual psychologists, ethologists and evolutionary biologists are quite mistaken, essentially the whole of my perceptual experience of the external world is unconsciously inferentially justified.

However, Huemer states also that "Sensory appearances then, provide noninferential justification for external world propositions." He appears to be resolving this apparent conflict by taking the position that he is only discussing epistemic beliefs and whether they are derived from perceptual experience by inferential or noninferential means, regardless of the means by which the perceptual experience comes into existence, whether this is directly or indirectly. He then argues that the naïve observer develops his beliefs about the external world noninferentially from his perceptual experience and contrasts this with the Indirect Realist position, which he claims would need to develop the same beliefs by inferential means.

I believe this is a straw man. I, like any other normal person, interpret what I see as literally what is there to be acted on without thinking and without needing to make any conscious inferences about it. There is of course no difference between the Direct Realist and the Indirect Realist, or even animals for that matter, in this regard. The difference arises in that I, as one of the rare humans who troubles himself with such notions, believe, when I bother to reflect on it, that when I look about me what appears to me as an external world is not actually the external world. I believe instead that I am actually looking at the inside of my conscious mind, and more specifically at an internal model of the environment produced and maintained from a multitude of influences by neural processes.

In other words, I have a set of beliefs about the external world, which are noninferentially derived (at least as regards their epistemology), and these include immediate, actionable beliefs such as "If I continue walking I will bump my nose on that wall." I apparently share this set of beliefs with all the other humans on the planet, and if we employ the usual behaviorist definitions of such things we will arrive also at the conclusion that animals share this set of beliefs. However, I think that this is a trivial truth, which proves nothing other than that we all have had essentially the same experiences from which we have learned to have expectations about what we perceive.

On the other hand I, as an Indirect Realist, have an additional set of beliefs, which are beliefs about the mechanism by which the first set of beliefs are created and maintained, and these beliefs are inferentially justified. In the first set of beliefs I fully believe that the appearance of a wall means I will bump my nose given certain actions, and I believe so without giving any thought to the ontological status of the appearance of the wall. In the second set of beliefs on the other hand I do not think that given our current theories of physics the notion of a physical world object "looking" like anything is even coherent, while the notion of a mental experience having a "look" is quite comprehensible. This second set of beliefs is about the ontological status of what appears to me, and is inferentially based on scientific evidence about the likely physical processes by which the appearances underlying the first set of beliefs are conveyed to my consciousness. In other words, the second, inferentially justified, set of beliefs are beliefs *about* the first set of beliefs. The two are entirely distinct and should not be conflated. There is thus a sense here in which we agree. That is, that the epistemology of ordinary, naïve, actionable, and perceptual beliefs are based on non-inferential justification from perceptual experience. Where we disagree is in whether or not this observation has anything to do with Indirect Realism.

1. ERNEST W. KENT'S COMMENTS ON PIERRE LE MORVAN

First let me thank Professor Le Morvan for this interesting and useful paper, which provides much-needed clarity concerning distinctions among the different Direct Realist positions available. What strikes me about it is that there are in fact so many minor variations that it becomes very difficult to mount any argument against "Direct Realism" as a concept since there is always another version, which the Direct Realist could offer that might escape it. In the same vein, counterexamples can be met with the criticism that even if correct they do not disprove that other perceptions are direct. One would prefer to be able to come to grips with a unique, central, Direct Realist concept. In the classification scheme presented here, "Ur-Direct Realism" as described in this paper now seems to be the most general case. This then is apparently what the Indirect Realist ought to be addressing.

Ur-Direct Realism's defining characteristic is stated to be that "… we perceive physical objects without a logically prior awareness of an objectified appearance." This then seems to be what the Indirect Realist must get a hold on to be certain of dealing with the issue at its root. I take "objectified appearance" to mean any representation of the object in any form other than the object itself, whether it be a bundle of light rays, a retinal image, a neural state, a sense datum, or any other phenomenal object other than awareness itself, however, awareness may be conceived (cf., e.g., Cairns, 2013, p.131) I take "logically prior awareness" in this case to refer to any awareness of such an intermediate representation that is a necessary precondition of perception.

Unfortunately, as Le Morvan points out, this is a negative definition and I am still left wondering what "direct" actually means as used by the Direct Realists. Perusing the various positions does not much clarify the issue. While they demarcate themselves from one another in various ways, they do not actually do much to explain in what sense they are "direct." I am left with the feeling that they frequently are using the term in quite different ways, and in most cases without a concrete notion of how it is supposed to work. Le Morvan provides some assistance where he can contrast them with Indirect Realist contenders, but on the whole when am I told, for example, that direct awareness consists of "a relation" with a distal object I do not feel in the least enlightened.

There are a number of possible meanings of "direct" evident in the positions reviewed in this work, which I will consider here. They fall into two broad categories:

1. The first possibility is that "direct" means that there exists some kind of link between awareness and the distal object that exists outside of the usual causal chain of light rays to retina, to neurons, to awareness. Let us examine this interpretation. (I limit myself to physical distal objects here. Le Morvan mentions some variants, which involve direct awareness of categories or ideals, but it would seem there is no basis on which even to speculate what that might actually mean.) The necessity of the links in the causal chain is well established. By altering it negatively or positively we can eliminate or produce sensations and perceptions. Is it possible that awareness nonetheless has some "direct" involvement with the distal object that is in addition to, and outside of, this chain, whether awareness requires the chain's existence or not?

It can be argued that of course we often (in fact always) do not perceive distal objects in a completely veridical manner since any number of intervening transformations can affect the image formed on the retina, or the neural activity resulting from it, etc., and hence our awareness must be of some objectified appearance instantiated by these intervening transformations. Further, interrupting this causal chain of intermediate representations eliminates perception of the object. Thus no matter what our awareness of the distal object is, it is mediated by these causally prior (logically prior in Le Morvan's terms) representations. However, Le Morvan (2004) instructs us that this conclusion does not invalidate Direct Realism because Direct Realism need not claim that direct awareness requires that objects appear exactly as they are, and hence our awareness may still be directly of the distal object even if (as he concedes) the intervening transformations and representations to which its image is subjected are causally responsible for it appearing as it does.

I take that to mean that, while our perceptions may be determined by and depend on the intermediate representations, we are not aware of them but, rather, are aware of the distal object "directly." Thus I assume there must be some sort of manner in which the distal object can have an effect on our awareness by this "direct" sort of connection with us.

The Indirect Realist is then placed in the position of having to demonstrate that the distal object *cannot* directly appear to the observer in a manner consistent with the intervening transformations of its representations by some influence outside of the causal chain of representations.

It is also argued that the distal object could not directly appear to us because we would then see it not as it is but as it was at some former time and it might not even still exist. However, Le Morvan (2004) again instructs us that this does not logically follow since Direct Realism need not claim that our direct awareness of the distal object is of the object as it is in the present and may be of it as it was at some past time. The Indirect Realist then has the additional burden of demonstrating that the distal object *cannot* "directly" appear to the observer in a manner consistent with the intervening transformations of its representations, even if our direct awareness may be of the object as it was at some past time.

I believe these things may in fact be demonstrated for all possible interpretations of "direct" that include *any* communication, influence, or connection between the distal object and the observer other than via the causal chain of intermediate representations. I make two assumptions. First, if a distal object appears X to an observer O, then unless O is hallucinating, a realist of any sort must conclude that *something* is appearing X to O or causing O to be in some state of awareness. Thus, if there is a direct link of any sort between the distal object and O, the distal object must be a causal participant in it. The Direct Realist must conclude that the distal object is what is appearing X to O since he denies that O is aware of anything else. The Indirect Realist may claim that some intervening representation in the causal chain is appearing X to O.

Second, as a realist, I assume the ordinary limitations of our current scientific understanding of the real world. No transfer of information faster than light, no precognition, no clairvoyant knowledge, etc. One could postulate endless nonphysical connections between the distal object and O, but such speculation contributes nothing unless there is some reason or evidence for hypothesizing the existence or nature of such a connection.

Let us then examine the possibility that awareness is "direct" exactly because there exists some kind of information-carrying link between awareness and the distal object that is outside of the usual causal chain of light rays to retina to neurons to awareness. I will attempt to show that this is not possible.

Let us suppose that although the causal chain of representations determines the appearance, the awareness is "direct" due to some other direct link, relation, effect, connection, participation, mutual understanding, etc., outside the ordinary causal chain. In that case, the critical events are any events in which a light ray from the distal object (or some subsequent neural state of affairs) is transformed by some means *en route* to O's awareness. The mere existence of the transformation in the path is not, by itself, a sufficient event. For example, if it were light passing through ripples in water, the ripples would have changed between the time the ray departed the distal object and the time it reached the water, or a filter may have been inserted after the ray departed. Thus at the time the ray departs the object, the object's necessary appearance is unknown at the location of the object. This information obviously must be present at the object for the object to manifest the correct appearance directly by *any* means. Thus this information must be transmitted to the location of the object, and this transmission must be initiated at the time and place of the transformation event.

There is always some transformation of the appearance of the distal object between it and O such as atmospheric absorption or scattering, insertion of a colored glass or deviating prism, etc., even if it is only the transformations produced by the inherent limitations of the eye and nervous system. It is simple to demonstrate that within the laws of physics it is quite impossible under any circumstances for both of two things to occur. One is that there is any information at the location of the distal object concerning what the transformed appearance X entails. The second is that any information whatever can reach the observer from the distal object before the object appearing X to O has already occurred. One or the other of these can be the case, but not both, and that is true even if the observer can be aware of the distal object as it was at an earlier time and regardless of any distances involved. The distal object appearing X to O directly by being a participant in some direct link outside the ordinary causal chain of representations contravenes the light speed limitation on transmission of information.

By the same arguments it can be shown that there is no physical information transfer possible concerning any change of state of O resulting from sensation produced through the ordinary causal chain that can allow the distal object to participate in any such direct interaction prior to its appearing X to O.

These things are true because, absent precognition, there can be no information at the distal object at the time a light ray departs it concerning what transformations may be encountered. Any information concerning what transformations of representation are encountered, or what changes of state they produce in O must then reach the object by some means originating at the point of such an encounter, or at O.

Suppose that the transformation is inserted at a random moment in time, t0. A light ray leaving the distal object will reach the transformation after some duration d1 and then reach the observer after a total duration of d2. Assuming current physics, under no circumstances can information about the state of O be available at the distal object before O's perceptual experience of the transformation occurs and the object appears X to O. This is because it would require a duration equal to (d2 − d1) for the causal change to reach O, and an additional duration equal to d2 for information about any change of state of O to reach the distal object, and $((d2 − d1) + d2) > (d2 − d1)$. Once such information arrives at the distal object it would take yet an additional duration equal to d2 for any resulting influence on O's awareness to reach O. It is thus physically impossible for the distal object to have any influence on itself appearing X to O prior to actually appearing X to O as a result of any change of state of O resulting from the insertion of the transformation.

The situation is identical with respect to information concerning any transformation *en route* interacting with the distal object if the transformation is inserted more than halfway from the distal object to O. In this case $(2 \times d1) > (d2 − d1)$ and information concerning the insertion of the transformation cannot reach the distal object before the object appears X to O, and again, an additional duration equal to d2 would then be required for it to have any resulting effect on its appearance to O.

If the transformation is inserted less than halfway from the distal object to X, then it is possible for information about the fact to reach the distal object prior to the object appearing X to O, but it is still not physically possible for any result of this to have any effect on the state of O prior to O's awareness of the object appearing X, since $((2 \times d1) + d2) > (d2 − d1)$.

Can the Direct Realist appeal to the state of the distal object at an earlier time than that of it appearing X to O? In the first two cases, clearly not since at any time prior to the object appearing X to O, information about the state of the transformation and the state of O is either incorrect or undefined at the location of the distal object. In the last case, there is a period extending from time $t0 + (2 \times d1)$ to time $t0 + d2$ during which information about the transformation has reached the distal object and before the distal object appears X to O. However, any influence of the distal object on O from any time in this interval would require a duration equal to d2 to reach O, and thus could not affect O prior to the object appearing X to O. Thus, even if O is allowed to have awareness of the distal object at any past time, there is no such past time before the object has already appeared X to O during which both that awareness could influence O and the distal object has information about the transformation.

It might be claimed that appearing X to O is a relational property of the distal object. That is, that the distal object has the property of appearing X if it is in a certain relation to O, such as appearing red if it is on the other side of a red filter from O. If this is a property of the object, then either it acquires this property when the relation is instantiated, in which case the same information transfer considerations already considered rule out its having any timely effect, or it requires that the object has had all possible properties for all possible relations *ab initio*. In the latter case, however, it cannot manifest the correct property until the nature of the relation is established, and this information cannot be present at the object at the time light departs it, so again the object cannot influence its appearance by any means other than the normal causal chain before it has already appeared X to O.

Even appeal to exotic physics such as quantum teleportation is of no avail since the instantaneous transfer of state in such effects still requires a prior, sublight speed transfer of the information to the remote partner in the experiment. It thus appears that a Direct Realist interpretation in the case of a transformation inserted at a random time into the light path from the distal object to O is not physically possible.

However, we may go further. One can generalize the situation and argue that there can never be any effective and timely fact of the matter at the object's location regarding how it is to appear to the observer. This is necessary because whether or not there exists at any instant a transformation of the appearance inserted subsequent to the object, one might be inserted after the light carrying the appearance of the object left the object. The two conditions, with and without an intervening transformation, are thus logically identical in terms of the inability of subsequent events in passage (including no event) or subsequent changes of state of the observer (including no change of state) to affect how the distal object appears to the observer via any mediation through the distal object. There is thus as little influence, either from the observer's state or the intermediate representations, able to affect the object's appearance to O in the nontransformed case as in the transformed case. If there is no transformation inserted and the perception is veridical, that can only be good luck unless the perception is indirect.

I thus argue that it is simply impossible with accepted physics for any state of the observer or any intermediate transformation (or non-transformation) of the appearance of the distal object to exert any influence on the distal object, which could cause it to appear X to O by any means the action of which on O preceded actual awareness of the appearance of X to O, if such means involve a "direct" link, relation, connection, participation, etc., outside the ordinary causal chain.

2. The second possibility we must consider is if there can be meanings of "direct," which apply to the situation where there is no interaction between the distal object and O other than through the normal causal chain.

First, there are versions of Direct Realism in which "direct" seems to be defined in terms of a state of the observer, for example, through what Brentano (1874/1973, Bk. 2, Ch. 1) terms "intentionality," or various abverbialist positions (e.g., Chisholm, 1957.) However, as we have seen in the above, no change of state of the observer can involve any causal interaction with the distal object outside of the chain of intermediate representations prior to it appearing X to O. Thus, either such a change of state is an awareness of some intermediate representation, or if it is not, saying that it is an awareness of the distal object is either incoherent or implies some unspecified mystical connection.

Next, it could be asserted that the property of the object appearing X to O is considered to be a property not of the object but of a relation between it and O, such as being so positioned that some transformation(s) occur (or do not occur) between them. The "bent stick" illusion seen through a glass of water is an example of such a relation. This is actually a tripartite relation, involving the positions of the distal object and O, and the presence or absence of the transformation(s) in the light path. It does not follow that direct awareness of such a property of the relation outside of the normal causal chain would constitute direct awareness of the object, and might better be considered as direct awareness of the intermediate representation following a transformation.

In any case, however, it is conceded that appearing X to O has an ontological commitment to the causal chain. This evolves over time as the wavefront encounters or fails to encounter transformations *en route* to O. The value of such a property of the relation is therefore not finally determined until the object has in fact appeared X to O since a further transformation might always occur. Neither are we aware of the appearance of the object evolving over time as the wavefront encounters successive transformations. Since the causal chain is logically and causally prior to the object appearing X to O, it follows that any such property of the relation is supervenient on, and subsequent to, the fact of the object finally appearing X to O, and any putative "direct" awareness of the property can have no effect on the object's appearance.

It seems possible on some readings that in fact all the Direct Realist really means is that he asserts that his awareness of the object is not a representation of it. Then, since his awareness is not numerically identical with any other representation, it is "direct" in the sense of not involving any representation at all. Of course he then can accept that it is still causally the result of the intermediate physical chain of transformed representations. I would argue (as I have elsewhere in this volume) that when "representation" is clearly defined in terms of veridical mappings from the information content inherent in the differential structure of the representation (physical or mental) to the distal object, then without question awareness itself is a representation. If it were not, then our awareness would have neither veridical intrinsic information nor differential structure, which obviously it does have. Thus awareness itself may be regarded as the final representation in the causal chain unless it is due to some "direct" connection outside of this chain, which I assert is physically impossible. If a Direct Realist argument then is in fact over whether or not to call awareness a representation, the whole discussion comes down to nothing more than an argument over what label to use for it, with no implied change in substance.

Finally, some approaches to Direct Realism seem to require something verging on the notion that the observer's perception itself is actually somehow in immediate contact with the distal object. Thus we have such phrases as, "...theories, which allow our cognitive powers to 'reach all the way to the objects themselves'" and so on. This seems to be very close to Naïve Realism and does not obviously allow for the perception to differ from the object. Beyond this, such ideas would seem to require that our perception is colocated in part with the object at the place and time at which it is exhibiting the properties perceived. This always requires that my current perception in the now also exists in part at some time in the past. This might be nanoseconds or thousands of years. I cannot imagine a coherent explanation of my perception existing thousands of years before I was born, even if we can allow a completely unknown mechanism for information transmission within this putative span of perception across space and time.

I have had to deal here with broad categories of Direct Realist positions, and I am sure that many will want to point to one distinction or another regarding particular theories. However, it seems clear that *no* Direct Realist theory has ever offered any account of how it is actually supposed to work. Even if we allow that the mechanism of the process is not yet understood, what evidence do we even have to suppose that there *is* such a process to explain in the first place? So far as I can see it is only that we seem to see things "out there" as if they were "out there" and we were immediately apprehending them. Of course this is true, but as support for existence of a "direct" process, this is nonsense. Modern neurobiology has developed and experimentally supported the concept of an internal model of the environment produced and maintained from a multitude of influences by neural processes. Our mental experience of this model, the lineal descendant of the old "sense-datum" idea, *ought* to look as if it were "out there." Why would we have evolved or learned any other experience of the input of our sensory apparatus than the one with the greatest predictive validity?

In sum, we have on the one hand the Direct Realist positions, currently without support from, nor testable hypotheses for, any scientific discipline, and on the other the Indirect Realist position, which is initially born out of physics and the neurosciences. It thus falls now to the Direct Realist either to produce an acceptable nonphysical means by which the object may appear directly to O or to show exactly how Direct Realism works within the context of current science. Simply applying labels is insufficient.

This criticism of Direct Realist shortcomings is of course not a criticism of Professor Le Morvan's paper, which has gone a good way toward clarifying for us the distinctions among the various subtheories. I can only hope that at some future date he may apply his evidently deep knowledge of the subject to a similar review of the possible mechanisms, which might be thought to underpin each of them.

ERNEST W. KENT'S COMMENTS ON FRED ADAMS

I enjoyed this paper and found it interesting. I was pleased to see the authors acknowledge the necessity of accepting the causal chain of sensory events, without which acknowledgment I think any Direct Realist theory is dead on arrival, and to see them identify, and propose an answer to, the subsequent problem of specifying which aspect of the causal chain of events is to be taken as the distal object of which we are to be directly aware; this kind of specificity of hypotheses is essential to furthering debate.

I will leave it to Bob French to comment on the remarks specific to his paper, but I have a few concerns about the general position from which they approach these issues. Since it seems we all accept that there are internal representations, that these form one part of the relation, and that they are the result of a physical causal chain beginning with the distal object and proceeding through neurological events and a (to-date nomic) causal connection to the phenomenal representation, how is it that we come to opposite conclusions regarding the "object of perception?" What else is there here that we might be understanding differently?

They assert in the introduction that, "*We think of perception … as a relation between internal mental events and external physical objects*.", and, "*The internal mental events are not the objects of perception but the perceivings of those external objects.*", and, "*The objects of perception are the physical objects and events in the world around us.*" In footnote one, they state, "*We accept that there are internal representations, but that they constitute one part of the perceptual relation to distal perceptual objects.*"

The intent here is clear. They mean that the distal object, directly and not through any intermediary, is what it is that I am perceiving. Their principle motivation for wanting to establish this conclusion seems similar to that of many other Direct Realists. They are impressed by the fact that our experience seems to be of objects "out there"; we seem to participate perceptually directly in an external world. Thus they say, "*When we experience the world, … we come into contact with the world.*", and again, "*We will defend the view that when the experiences are veridical and of the world, the world itself is on the other end.*"

They also embrace the physical causal chain of events leading to neural states of affairs and agree that, "*On this view, qualitative states of mind are representations. When of external objects, the qualitative states of mind arise because various areas of the brain have been recruited to represent types of external properties of objects and events.*" Then they assert that something in addition to the information available through the causal chain is available to perception by virtue of the internal representation standing in a relation to a real object "out there." Thus, they say, "*Matt's tactile perception consists of this relation between the external source of his perceptual experiences (the keys on the keypad itself) and the internal mental perceivings that constitute Matt's part of the perceptual relation…*," and, "*Yet the qualia of the experience is not solely due to the neurochemical properties in the brain, but rather to these neural properties and activations standing in a representational relationship to their external causes.*", and, "*...on this view this means that qualia are not reducible to the neural chemical properties of neural events alone because they are representations. Representations are of/about things and this is not merely a neuro-chemical matter....*"

They appeal to correlation to explain how a particular representation is identified (and if "correlation" is a stand-in for some much more complicated information processing I have no quarrel with that.) They then seem to suggest that this somehow allows experience to "jump across" the other steps in the causal chain directly to the object represented. They define the distal object as the one "best correlated" with the experience. There will certainly be some distal cause with which the experience could be best correlated, and they are free to define the two as being related by that fact. However, this does not provide any new means of conveying to the phenomenal experience information about the distal cause to which it is so correlated.

Here we part ways. I want to know whether the information in the neural state of affairs does or does not contain all of the information necessary for the phenomenal experience. If it does, then why do we need something else? If it does not, and they say it does not, then where else can additional information in the phenomenal experience come from? The only option would seem to be from the "relation" they posit. When they say that explaining the full nature of the qualia requires, "*these neural properties and activations standing in a representational relationship to their external causes.*" What does this mean?

If it means something that is *not* already encoded in the causal chain terminating in a representation by the neural state, including any representation of physical relations to external objects, then I want to know by what other route it gets to the phenomenal experience. If the information *is* already provided via the causal chain including the neural state, then I want to know what "direct" is supposed to mean and why there is any reason for using the word.

If the relation is bringing something additional to the perception that is not mediated by the "neurochemical properties of the brain," the information needs some physical substrate for transmission. Since the neurochemical events, which they claim are inadequate are the end result of the physical causal chain, how does a "relation" causally affect a perception outside of this physical causal chain? Since calling it a "relation" tells nothing at all,

I assume they mean to say that the perception and the distal object are "related" by *some* causal process, but it appears to be one, which "directly" links the internal representation to the distal object without going through the brain. This begins to sound as if they are flirting with mysticism.

Perhaps they are saying that there is information that is *not* in the internal representation that is mediated by the neurochemical events, but rather is something that my perceptual state reaches out to find directly in the external world. But again, we have the same issue. By what physical mechanism does this clairvoyance accomplish this outside of what is already fully accounted for in the causal chain and neurochemical processes that they have already embraced but labeled inadequate?

Perhaps they are only trying to say that something like the correlation process they describe for uniquely identifying the external object, or perhaps prior knowledge of how things are in the external world, or understanding of the situation context, or all of these are needed in addition to the instantaneous state of the causal chain of neural activation to give a perception of the world "as it is, out there." Of course this would be true, but nonetheless it all has to come down to neural activity somehow via physical means unless they are aware of some nonphysical means for this additional information from the external world to get in, or for perception to get out to it. Further, the result of these other factors must be locally represented in neural states, by encoding information stored from prior sensory events or otherwise generated by brain processes, and incorporated into the current state responsible for the current phenomenal experience unless they can suggest how a direct relation from the physical object to the phenomenal experience can transfer information in some other manner.

Consider, for example, their rebuttal to the bent stick argument. They assert that what Jill really sees is a straight stick appearing bent. If this is true and is due to a direct relation to the unbent stick, then Jill really is perceiving the stick directly but, because there is a refractive medium interposed in her line of sight, there is *no way* that this direct relation can be mediated by any physical causal chain. Either her object of perception is a neural representation of a bent stick reflecting the bent stick image on her retina, or her object of perception is the straight stick appearing bent directly by nonphysical means.

However, this may be (and I am sure they really do have some nonmystical interpretation of what they are saying) it is clear that they do not think that the perception of the object as it is, "out there," is already a property of the phenomenal experience, preconsciously produced by neural processes, but must require something else in the form of an additional relation to explain our experience of the world. It seems to me that they are at least implicitly applying a view of neural processing, which fails to take into account modern concepts of internal world modeling, motor feedforward, control theoretic concepts, and other features of current neuroscience. As a result, their view of neural sensory processing very naturally falls short of producing the picture of the world they want. Their answer to this shortcoming, however, is to posit a "relation" to the external world to provide what is missing. On the contrary, the currently accepted view of most neurobiologists is that the brain maintains an internal model of the environment produced and updated from a multitude of influences by neural processes. That is, that there is a neural model of the environment, that this model is that of which we are aware, and that it is continuously servoed to the best fit between current sensory input, predictions of sensory effects resulting from commanded body actions, knowledge and beliefs about the current state of the environment, including illumination and other factors. Neural mechanisms of computation are thought to achieve this according to the usual algorithms of control theory. Servoing the model to the sensory input plus a variety of other information sources, and then servoing the output of the system to the best-fit model is standard practice for control systems from brains to robots to oil refineries (see, e.g., Kent and Albus, 1984 for a concept overview.).

Among the other sources of information used to instantiate the model will be mechanisms for locating the represented object in space in three dimensions (of which there are many in addition to binocular vision) and for converting that into the conative space of actions through metric transformations, learned from birth, which transform between visual space and kinesthetic and proprioceptive space and which, in addition to guiding action, provide feedforward to the model to predict and filter out image motion due to intended actions. At the same time, processes in the multiple visual areas of the brain are adding object details. Predicted visual features are used to improve noise rejection and recognition and tracking of incoming sensory data. Kalman filtering and predictive modeling are used to generate expectations of multimodal sensory data that are differenced with incoming signals to allow optimal control of the model parameters in the face of noisy and incomplete input. The internal model thus gets additional information over and above retinal and other sensory surface input added to it concerning the location and nature of each object in it through *preconscious* processes that operate *before* it is presented to awareness. If you want to see this in action, please try the little experiment with the folded paper and pencil in Appendix A of Chapter 4 in the current volume; it's fun.

They align their views with authors such as Dretske (1981), and it is worth noting that the above view of neural information processing used to servo internal models has much in common in principle with his "informational" view of perceptual processing, which he contrasts with the "causal" view (op. cit., p. 157.) However, this is neutral with regard to the object of perception. Dretske identifies a "primary representation," which he asserts is the representation of the distal object best correlated with experience. This, however, is not in any conflict with the idea that the object of perception is an internal neural model of the world, including the "principal representation" represented as such, together with its location in a phenomenal model of the world (among its other multimodal properties).

He remarks (Dretske op. cit., p. 163) that we perceive the external world as staying still despite the fact that the retinal image moves as we move our eyes (and this is also true when we turn our head, or even turn somersaults). He also notes that we do perceive motion when we track a moving object with our eyes and it stays still on the retinal image. However, in 5 s you can demonstrate the error in his conclusion: close one eye, place your finger on the lid of the open eye at the corner, and jiggle your eyeball. The world moves! What is happening here is that ordinarily the motor cortex provides feedforward to the internal model, which predicts and cancels out the expected effects of bodily motion on the retinal image as it produces its updated best model of the environment. However, it has only evolved connections for supporting this for the types of induced retinal motion that move the image around in the course of ordinary bodily actions. Anything out of the ordinary such as jiggling the eye makes the world seem to move with the retinal image, which is just what Dretske is arguing would be the case if we were *not* perceiving the distal object directly.

He proposes constancy effects as argument that our perception is of the distal object and not the details of the retinal projection, but of course constancy effects fail when, for example, the true nature of the light source is hidden from the observer. This is exactly as would be expected of an internal model servoed to, among other things, knowledge of the illumination. He is correct that it is not the details of the retinal projection (alone) that determine what we perceive, but this in no way implies that our apparent perception of the distal object is not in fact perception of an internal model of it.

Thus, if Adams et al. intend that their additional relation is physical but consists of an augmentation of the basic sensory causal chain by some object selection such as through the correlation they mention and/or other additions to the phenomenal presentation of the bare retinal image, then yes, something conceptually similar to that happens, or at least one of its distant modern descendants does. That has nothing to do with a direct relation, however. My claim is that:

1. Perceptual experience is the result of the brain's maintenance of an internal model of the world as described above and requires no relation to the external object beyond that of the physical sensory causal chain plus a (currently nomic) causal dependence of the content of awareness on proximal neural events encoding this model.

2. That this internal representation is *complete* in the sense that it presents as immediate phenomenal experience all of the phenomenal properties of the object that Adams et al. assert would require an additional relation to the external object.

In other words, my phenomenal experience of the object's "out-there-ness" is just that. It is a phenomenal property no different than it being yellow and no differently produced. It is the result of an information processing problem solved in the brain preconsciously, and the solution is made part of the internal representation, right along with the color of the object and other phenomenal data. Our experience of its location in external space, for example, is a phenomenal experience that requires nothing beyond ordinary neural processes to account for it.

Here then is our second point of departure. I view the properties which constitute my perception of the world as "out there" to be not only wholly phenomenal in character but also in fact absolutely unlike the physical world in substance, and to have only a mathematical mapping relationship to its properties. The object's physical property of being "out there" must not be confused with my phenomenal experience of "out-there-ness." Looking like something is not a property of the physical world; it is a property of the phenomenal experience. Physical substance does not "look" like anything; it has properties, but they are not phenomenal properties. To confuse the object's physical property of being "out there" with our phenomenal experience of its "out-there-ness" is a category error. This is the same error one would be making if they confused our experience of yellow with the physical object's preferential wavelength reflectivity. They would be confusing the mental and the physical. As a result I find the concept of "direct" experience of physical objects impossible. Adams et al. do not appear to go this far in that they do consider the perception to be entirely phenomenal in character, I believe, but nonetheless their direct relation between the physical external object and phenomenal immediate experience is problematic in that, absent any other explanation of its nature, it seems to be only a mask behind which just such an identification of physics and phenomenal experience hides and by which phenomenal properties are ascribed to physical objects.

Viewed from the perspective of a robust neural process for generating a full phenomenal account of the world's appearance, the motivation for inexplicable additional relations vanishes. Yet, rejection of the notion that as we look around us we are actually looking at the insides of our minds rather than at an external world is so deeply rooted that some (e.g., Allston, 1999) have even proposed *literally* inexplicable (i.e., in principle ontologically irreducible) relations to preserve the conceit of apprehending external reality directly "as it is."

Dretske (1981, p. 162) appears to be falling into this trap when he tries to explain why we do not experience hearing our tympanic membrane rather than the bell, and of course we seemingly do not experience hearing our auditory membrane or seeing our visual cortex activity as such in any way we would recognize. However, he is making the *assumption* that we are *not* in fact hearing and seeing *exactly* those things, whereas of course what we see and hear can just as well be precisely how we experience those items. If he assumes this because our experiences seem unlike those objects, one wonders why he then has no problem with them seeming unlike the electrical bonds in the distal objects that are the source of the information reaching our receptors. In the same way, he argues that the brain's way of coding perceptual objects usually puts the object outside the organism, and this is true, but it in no way implies that what we are perceiving is not an internal model of the external object including, as above, its modeled spatial location.

In general, once it is understood that the neurobiology involves something more complex than a simple encoding of the retinal image into a phenomenal representation, arguments often advanced in favor of direct perception of the distal object turn out to be better explained by the object of perception being a servoed neural model of the world.

Against my position it might be argued that since our understanding of the causal dependence of our phenomenal experience on our neural processes is currently only of a nomic nature, it is in fact logically no better than a claim of a direct dependence on all the physical objects of the world directly. Strictly speaking, this is true, but in reality the difference between the two is enormous. We have every reason to believe that there is a special relationship between our phenomenal experience and neural tissue. We know that these phenomenal properties can be evoked or altered by direct neural stimulation in a lawful and predictable manner. We can record changes in neural activity contingent on phenomenal events when the underlying stimulus is constant (Kommeier and Bach, 2012). We do not yet have an understanding of the mechanism by which this occurs, but it is at least possible to make plausible and testable hypotheses (e.g., Penrose, 1994). Nothing of the sort is true of a direct relation between phenomenal experience and other ordinary objects of physics.

In summary, I find no support for the authors' contention that anything in our phenomenal experience of the world requires the assumption of anything other than the object of perception being the internal world model maintained by the nervous system from, among much else, current sensory input. On the contrary, there are no sustainable arguments for supposing that our phenomenal experience of the world is not in total "of and about" our "neural properties and activations." Thus I assert that the assumption of a direct relation to physical objects is unnecessary. It is also highly problematic in terms of causal mechanisms of information transfer.

STEVEN LEHAR'S COMMENTS ON MICHAEL HUEMER'S THE VIRTUES OF DIRECT REALISM

Huemer makes a reasonable case for believing that your foot is really there when you see it. He calls it a "noninferential justification": you do not have to prove that your foot is there, you can see directly that it is there just by looking. No inference is required, the observation is direct. But what Huemer ignores is the *basis* for that justification, and that basis is the three-dimensional visual experience that you have when you see your foot. But Huemer misidentifies his experience of his foot for the foot itself, which he claims to be able to see directly, but Huemer never explains how the image of his foot ever enters his experience in the first place, he simply assumes that perception is direct, without ever explaining how. Just as you know with absolute certainty that your foot is right there where you see it, a similar "noninferential justification" confirms that perception of your foot is direct. You can see it right there before you, so that demonstrates that you can see things out in the world directly. The entire theory of Direct Perception is itself a "noninferential justification" of the directness of perception confirmed by direct observation and nothing else.

1. STEPHEN LEHAR'S COMMENTS ON MICHAEL HUEMER

According to Phenomenal Conservatism, appearances are an intrinsic, ultimate source of justification. In the absence of defeaters, the appearance that P suffices for P to be justified, and no further beliefs, awareness, or other mental states are required. ...it simply is rational to start from the way things seem, by default. Sensory appearances, then, provide non-inferential justification for external-world propositions. [Emphasis *added*]

But sensory appearances can be deceiving, most clearly in the case of dreams and hallucinations, so they can hardly serve as an ultimate source of justification for anything except for the existence of the experience itself, as it is experienced to be. Illusory experience clearly demonstrates that experience is not the same as reality.

But the debate on this issue is hampered not only by the use of different terms and terminology by the two sides but also by profoundly different conceptualizations of the issue and the entities involved, with the result that the two sides argue at cross-purposes due to a failure to reach consensus on what the debate is actually about. Fig. 13.9.1 illustrates the paradigmatic divide with the example of the experience of your own foot. Fig. 13.9.1A–C depicts the theory of indirect perception, from A: the objective external foot, through B: the subjective experience of that foot (with eyes open if the foot is in your visual field), to C: (if you think about it) the cognitive inference that *there is a foot.* Fig. 13.9.1D–F depicts the theory of direct perception.

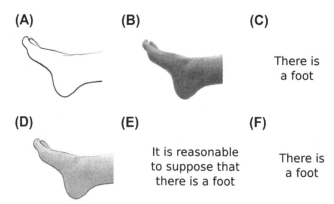

Figure 13.9.1 The paradigmatic divide. Indirect perception: (A) The objective physical foot. (B) The subjective experience of the foot (sense data). (C) The inference. Direct perception: (D) The objective/subjective foot. (E) Noninferential justification. (F) The inference.

The key difference is that D represents a superposition of items A and B into a single objective/subjective entity that is somehow both the objective external foot and also the subjective experience of that foot. Huemer would object vehemently to calling item D in any way a subjective experience, but the three-dimensional colored surface of the experienced foot is an essential aspect of experience that cannot so easily be dismissed as part of experience.

The problem with merging these two totally dissimilar entities (one a physical object outside your head, the other a spatial experience arguably within it) is that they have different characteristics: One is a real volume of living tissue complete to every molecule and atom at virtually infinite resolution, the other is a cartoon-like sketch of only the exposed surfaces at much reduced resolution: the hidden volume and hidden rear surfaces are not experienced directly, as are the surfaces exposed to view. And the resolution of experience falls far short of the molecular, or even the cellular scale. The resolution of experience is limited by the optical limitations of the eye, as received indirectly through sensory processing, not by the limitations of actual reality perceived directly out in the world. If perception were direct, we would perceive the internal volume and tissues of our foot, not just its surfaces that are exposed to an open eye.

Furthermore, the objective external foot and the internal experience of your foot are easily distinguishable by simply closing one's eyes. The part of the world that blinks out of existence (the entire visual field!) when you blink is the internal world of experience causally downstream of your closing eyelids, while the item that continues to exist uninterrupted by the closing of your eyelids is the objective external foot. How can the one disappear in a blink while the other continues to exist uninterrupted, if there is no distinction between them in D? Clearly the very concept of the objective/subjective structure is a direct expression of the Naïve Realist assumption that what you see is what is out there and captures the paradox of its very nature in the model itself. The union of these dissimilar entities into a single concept represents a category error at the most profound level.

What Huemer is really arguing is that the item B, the sense data of visuospatial experience, is somehow impossible in principle, and therefore he replaces it with E: a nonspatial "justification" based on nothing other than the direct observation of the foot out in the world D, the impossible objective/subjective entity that defies causal explanation. Huemer dutifully reformulates the theory of Indirect Perception with the image-like sense data surgically removed, before destroying it as a model with an essential component missing. The missing component is the one he removes.

In his characterization of the theory of Indirect Realism Huemer describes sense data as if they were *inferential justifications* for external world propositions, i.e., an intermediate hypothesis between the direct visual experience of the world and our inferences based on those experiences, i.e., item E in the diagram. He claims that the Indirect Realist, on seeing his own foot, is not satisfied with the mere direct perception of his foot (item D) but requires an intermediate *noninferential justification* (item E) for the obvious presence of his foot before he can conclude that "there is a foot," (item F) an inference based on direct observation. What this view is missing is that the "noninferential justification" is the sense data themselves, item B, and they are image-like by their nature, not at all like cognitive inferences drawn from them. Huemer is right, there is no need for an intermediate inference, the visuospatial experience is evidence enough for the presence of the foot. But Huemer falls victim to the grand illusion of visual experience and believes that he can see his foot directly, bypassing the mediation of his senses.

Huemer explains that when an Indirect Realist observes their own foot, "my justification for believing that the foot exists depends upon my having justification for some other beliefs. What other beliefs? ...one or more propositions about mind-dependent phenomena – sensations, 'sense data,' states of being appeared to, etc.," (item E in the diagram).

No it does not depend on *propositions* about "sense data": It depends on the presence in our experience of the sense data themselves, an item that requires no propositions to verify its presence, it is perceived directly, where it exists in our mind, presumably represented in some form in our brain. While it is incredible to propose direct experience of objects outside of the mind and brain where there is no computational or representational mechanism, it is perfectly reasonable to propose direct experience of representations within the mind and brain. Indeed, experience would not be possible if we could not experience the internal states of our own brain, directly, because our mind *is* those internal states.

The reason Huemer has difficulty identifying the sense data of experience is because he misidentifies them as the actual objective foot itself, beyond the sensory surface, the impossible item D in the diagram, and thus his idea of an observation of this direct experience is like item E, a cognitive "justification," not a spatial image, a "justification" that depends on the objective external foot, observed directly out where it lies in D. Huemer never explains how real-world information enters into subjective experience beyond the statement that it is self-evident that it does, despite the obviously indirect and representational nature of the sensory path through eye, optic nerve, and brain, not to mention visual after-images and propagation delays.

Later Huemer argues that, for example, when a normal person sees a marmot, he does not go through anything like the reasoning: "Well, I'm having a marmot-representing sensory experience right now. I wonder what could be causing it. Let me list the alternative explanations and the theoretical virtues and vices of each ... Okay, it looks like the real-world theory wins out. So there is most likely an actual marmot in front of me." The chain of reasoning that Huemer denies corresponds to the entity E that he added himself as a replacement for item B, the sense data of experience, the "marmot-representing sensory experience" that is very similar to the experience had when viewing this picture:

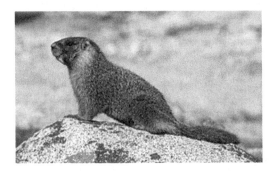

It is *this* image-like entity whose very existence Huemer denies, confusing it instead for a direct experience of a marmot out in the world (or in this case, of the picture of a marmot out on the page), denying the existence of the intermediate representation, the one that goes dark when you close your eyes. Tellingly, Huemer does not argue that sense data cannot exist; he merely argues that it is self-evident that perception is direct, with no intermediate representation required.

Huemer does not engage in a debate between Direct and Indirect Perception but simply declares victory from the outset, the debate is already over! The conclusion is self-evident!

> *The Direct Realist ... has no problem granting external-world knowledge to typical adults, as well as children and animals. On my account, the justification for external-world propositions* derives directly from appearances, with no auxiliary premises needed. *To have a justified belief that my left foot exists, all I have to do is have an experience in which the foot seems to me to exist, with no reasons for doubting its existence, and that experience must cause me to think the foot exists.* [Emphasis *added*]

Huemer argues that the existence of illusory experience, such as dreams and hallucinations, does not cast doubt on veridical perception when it is not illusory, for the same reason that you can be sure that your foot is really there where you see it. But Huemer misses the central point: The very fact that the visual system is *capable* of constructing illusory worlds of experience is direct evidence for the sense data, item B in the paradigmatic diagram, whose very existence Huemer denies. A hallucinated scene is composed exclusively of raw sense data, and its very existence demonstrates that it is possible to have an extended visuospatial experience of objects that do not actually exist. Therefore sense data *can* and *do* exist, and thus it is perfectly possible (indeed inescapably obvious) that the sense data of our experience are indeed a construct of our brain causally downstream of our eyelids and retinae, and that is why they exhibit perspective projection, and why they go dark when we close our eyes.

Huemer further raises what he calls the Symmetry Argument as an argument for Indirect Perception that he finds "theoretically fishy".

That is, the view that the Indirect Realist takes of sensory appearances is not one that he could take about appearances in general, but there is no obvious reason why sensory appearances should be epistemologically different from non-sensory appearances. The most theoretically natural approach would treat sensory and non-sensory appearances alike, as Direct Realists do. [Emphasis added]

Again, this argument is only cogent from a Direct Realist perspective. What Huemer is saying is that entity E in his version of Indirect Realism is no different epistemologically from a regular inference such as F in the diagram, that is, he sees no obvious difference between a "sensory appearance" like E, and a nonsensory one like F. Of course what Huemer is missing is that a sensory appearance is actually more like B, an explicit spatial image rather than a cognitive proposition, and a spatial image in experience is clearly different epistemologically from a nonsensory proposition such as "it is reasonable to suppose there is a foot."

As to the question of how facts about the world can enter our experience, but for the obvious route through our senses, Huemer states that they obviously do, perception is self-evidently direct, at least when perception is not illusory, and that is enough for him. It is not persuasive for those not already persuaded.

The theory of Direct Perception is nothing other than an elaborate rationalization of Naïve Realism, the persistent conviction that one can see the world directly, out where it lies, against all of the obvious evidence of the representational architecture from the eye through the optic nerve to the brain. What is curious about this debate is that proponents of Direct Perception do not consider the possibility of sense data interposed between the world and their experience of it, they reject that notion out of hand at the outset, as self-evidently untrue, based on the "obvious" directness of perception (when it is not illusory or hallucinatory). Huemer cannot conceptualize the model ABC in the paradigmatic diagram, he gets a headache thinking about item B, the sense data as an image-like experience, he has no idea what that could possibly be because it corresponds to nothing in his (direct) experience of the world DEF, so he replaces it in his mind with the closest thing he can conceptualize, item E, a kind of "observation" of the objective world, observed directly in D, where an "observation" is a cognitive state: there is no image in experience, no sense data, or extended spatial experience. Experience is not a spatial structure, it is an observational state. Except in dreams and hallucinations where a spatial structure appears in experience in the absence of any object to be experienced directly, but that is to be ignored, it is not relevant to normal perception.

2. CONCLUSION

The debate between direct and indirect perception is clearly a paradigm debate, in the sense that the opposing views use different characterizations of the facts of the case, which makes agreement pretty much impossible. Proponents of Direct Perception argue that paradigm ABC is impossible in principle, whereas proponents of Indirect Perception argue that it is DEF, which is impossible in principle. The key item that distinguishes the two paradigms is item B, as contrasted with item D. Is it possible that the sense data of experience, the three-dimensional world that we experience with eyes open, is an intermediate representation B? Or is our view of the world direct, unmediated by sense data as in D? The answer can be found quite simply by closing one's eyes. But, the Direct Realist will object, closing your eyes does not change the spatial image in D, the objective external object itself, it merely closes off access to that direct view of the world, the world continues to exist in D, it is just that our experience of it goes dark in E. This is not a rejection of the Indirect Realist view of perception as ABC, it is merely an alternative explanation of the same facts by way of DEF, the only problem being that paradoxical impossible entity D, the objective/subjective foot, and the embarrassing evidence of dreams and hallucinations. What actually happens to entity D when we blink our eyes open and closed? When they are open, we see the foot directly, out where it lies, where our experience of the foot is of a three-dimensional structure. With eyes closed the structure disappears, while continuing to exist as a 3D structure. In other words item D continues to exist uninterrupted, but item E loses access to it and thus our awareness is confined to E. How can that be? If perception is direct, then how can our eyelids block that direct perception? The answer provided by the theory of Direct Perception seems to be "I don't know how, but obviously it does!" The directness of perception is as self-evidently true as is the existence of my foot where I see it now. To which the only cogent reply is: Until you blink. The real foot continues to exist, your visual experience of it does not. The indirectness of perception is as sure as the blink of your eyes. Epistemologically speaking, item B, our subjective experience of the world is the only thing we can ever know with any certainty to actually exist, whether real, as in veridical perception, or illusory as in dreams and hallucinations. The theory of Direct Perception turns epistemology on its head and asks us to doubt the existence of item B, the only thing we can be absolutely certain to exist, which is our own conscious experience *as we experience it*. There is no deeper category error over the question of what is real and what is not.

REFERENCES

Allston, W., 1999. Back to the theory of appearing. Philos. Perspect. 13, 181–203.
Austin, J., 1962. Sense and Sensibilia. Oxford University Press, Oxford.
Brentano, F., 1874/1973. Psychologie vom Empirischen Standpunkte. Dunker and Humbolt, Leipzig. Psychology from an Empirical Standpoint, 1973, Routledge, London.
Cairns, D., 2013. The Philosophy of Edmund Husserl. Springer, Dordrecht.
Chisholm, R., 1957. Perceiving: A Philosophical Study. Cornell University Press.
Dennett, D., 1991. Consciousness Explained. Little Brown, Boston.
Dretske, F., 1995. Naturalizing the Mind. MIT Press, Cambridge.
Dretske, F., 1981. Knowledge and the Flow of Information. MIT Press/Bradford, Cambridge, M.A.
Duhem, P., 1906/1954. The Aim and Structure of Physical Theory. Princeton University Press, Princeton.
Fish, W., 2009. Perception, Hallucination, and Illusion. Clardenon Press, Oxford.
Gettier, E., 1963. Is justified true belief knowledge? Analysis 23, 121–123.
Goldman, A., 1979. What is justified belief? In: Pappas, G. (Ed.), Justification and Knowledge. D. Reidel, Dordrecht, pp. 1–23.
James, W., 1890. Principles of Psychology. Henry Holt, New York.
James, W., 1904. Does 'consciousness' exist? J. Philos. Psychol. Sci. Methods 1, 481–491.
Kent, E., Albus, J., 1984. Servoed world models as interfaces between robot control systems and sensory data. Robotica 1984 (2), 7–25.
Kommeier, J., Bach, M., 22 March, 2012. Frontiers in Human Neuroscience.
Krauskopf, J., 1963. Effect of retinal stabilization on the appearance of heterochromatic targets. J. Opt. Soc. Am. 53, 741–744.

Lakatos, I., 1970. Falsification and the methodology of scientific research programmes. In: Lakatos, I., Musgrave, A. (Eds.), Criticism and the Growth of Knowledge. Cambridge University Press, Cambridge.

Le Morvan, P., July 2004. Arguments against direct realism and how to counter them. Am. Philos. Q. 41 (3).

McDowell, J., 1982/2009. Criticism, defeasability, and knowledge. In: Byrne, A., Logue, H. (Eds.), Disjunctivism: Contemporary Readings. MIT Press, Cambridge.

Moore, G., 1959. A defence of common sense. In: Moore, G. (Ed.), Philosophical Papers. George Allen and Unwin, London, pp. 32–59.

Penrose, R., 1994. Shadows of the Mind: A Search for the Missing Science of Consciousness. Oxford University Press.

Popper, K., 1972. Objective Knowledge. Oxford University Press, Oxford.

Quine, W., 1951. Two dogmas of empiricism. Philos. Rev. 60, 20–43.

Reid, T., 1764/1970. Inquiry into the Human Mind. University of Chicago Press, Chicago.

Reid, T., 1785/1969. Essays on the Intellectual Powers of Man. MIT Press, Cambridge.

Russell, B., 1912. The Problems of Philosophy. Henry Holt, New York.

Russell, B., 1921. The Analysis of Mind. George Allen and Unwin, London.

Russell, B., 1927. The Analysis of Matter. Kegan Paul, London.

Russell, B., 1940. An Inquiry into Meaning and Truth. George Allen and Unwin, London.

Russell, B., 1948. Human Knowledge its Scope and Limits. 1948, George Allen and Unwin, London.

Smythies, J., 1994. The Walls of Plato's Cave. Avebury, Aldershot.

Tye, M., 1995. Ten Problems of Consciousness a Representational Theory of the Phenomenal Mind. MIT Press, Cambridge.

Wittgenstein, L., 1953. Philosophical Investigations. Macmillan, New York.

Wright, E., 2008. The Case for Qualia. MIT Press, Cambridge.

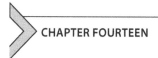

CHAPTER FOURTEEN

Rebuttals by Indirect Realists

Robert French
Adjunct Instructor, Philosophy, Oakland Community College, Waterford Township, MI, United States

JOHN SMYTHIES REPLY TO EVA SCHMIDT[1]

Schmidt has presented some well-crafted arguments against the concepts of the block universe, a moving time, and the geometrical and topological relations between physical space and phenomenal space, as I presented these in my chapter. However, I do not accept any of her counterarguments. Alas, to further this interesting debate properly would require far more space than is available here. So I refer the reader to my book "The Walls of Plato's Cave" that covers these points thoroughly.

I will therefore concentrate on her second theme—how activity in brain mechanisms brings about our seeing external objects. Here some new and important experimental neuroscientific evidence has recently been obtained that strongly supports the indirect theory.

The first set of evidence deals with the role of virtual reality mechanisms in vision. The Direct Realist theory supposes that vision allows us to see what is actually "out there"—barring some well-documented visual illusions and the occasional hallucination. However, this turns out not to be the case. The primary visual cortex V1 (which plays a key role in conscious vision) gets only 10% of its neuronal input from the retina (mainly foveal) and 90% (mainly peripheral) from higher sensory cortex. Thus 10% of what we see reports what is actually "out there," whereas the other 90% reports what the brain computes to be most probably "out there"—which constitutes virtual reality. As Francis Crick put it "What you see is not what is really there; it is what your brain believes is there." More details of how this is done have recently been discovered. This brings in the second concept relevant to vision, which is information compression. The relevance of this is as follows.

The brain is faced with a never-ending flood of information coming in over its sensory input, much of which is redundant as far as efficient

---

[1] I would like to thank Pierre Le Morvan and Eva Schmidt for their insightful comments on my paper. I address the remarks separately except for where there is an overlap; in which case I address the remarks together.

Direct versus Indirect Realism
ISBN 978-0-12-812141-2
https://doi.org/10.1016/B978-0-12-812141-2.00014-3
241

information processing relevant to action and memory formation is concerned. In particular, changes in informant input that are important tend to be located in the fovea, where attention is focused, whereas information on what happens in the periphery of vision is usually mainly redundant. To process the entire input would lead to a colossal waste of precious computational resources. So the brain has developed the following mechanism (Smythies, 2017; Smythies and d'Oreye de Lantrmange, 2016). Higher visual cortex has a powerful retrograde projection to V1 where it forms a "map" overlying the "map" of "what is out there" mediated by the input to V1 from the retina. The input from the higher cortex carries information of what the brain predicts to be "out there." In V1 cortex these two maps are superimposed, and, where the information is the same in both maps, the item is deleted. Thus only what is new gets transmitted from V1 to higher sensory cortex where it attracts attention and further processing. This compressed, and thus more efficient, computational process results in a change in what we see that takes in the change(s).

Interestingly digital television uses very much the same mechanism. The first frame of a series received in a TV transmission is passed "as is" to higher centers where its contained information is processed so as to produce the correct picture on the TV screen. However, in the next and subsequent frames only differences between a frame and the previous frame are transmitted to higher centers. This results in a very great saving of expensive computational resources.

I suggest that the discovery that the brain uses extensively both virtual reality and information compression technologies poses difficulties for the Direct Realist theory, which does not allow from such process to occur in its account of how seeing operates. The theory states that we see directly what is really "out there"—not that we see mainly what the brain computes is most probably "out there."

DAVID MCGRAW'S REPLY TO EVA SCHMIDT

Professor Schmidt speaks of my (alleged) claim "that we become aware of things in the world and their properties only via our contact with the phenomenal qualities of intra-mental impressions." Then she suggests that I give up this claim in favor of full direct realism.

Now, direct realism might perhaps be the better answer if the only alternative were that people become aware of things via their contact with impressions. Then again, even given direct realism, there would still be the further question of whether direct realism could be reconciled with materialism.

But in fact, I did not say, and do not believe, that people become aware of things via their contact with impressions. What I said was that the perceptual impression in the mind *is already* some sort of awareness of the real thing in the real world. Along this line, of course I say "the processes going on in the perceptual system are not something that obstructs the perceiver's contact with her surroundings." These processes lead up to the impression in the mind, and this impression constitutes the awareness, and so the processes are the *means by which* one has contact with the world, not an obstruction. Again, one's impressions acquired through the senses do not *mediate* one's perceptions—they *are* the perceptions.

In what way does this answer differ from direct realism? Perceptual impressions in the mind have their own distinctive character as things within the mind. This character is what is meant in speaking of the phenomenal as opposed to the physical. In what way, if any, does the phenomenal line up with the physical when sensory experience is veridical? On the view here, only the kind of correspondence described in the essay is required. But direct realism affirms a much stronger view of matching or similarity.

This stronger claim is very questionable, but that point may be left aside for the moment. Even if this stronger claim were true, it would be contrary to materialism. That is the central claim of the essay.

Remarkably, what all this involves can be illustrated by something Professor Schmidt takes to be opposed to what I said. "[Direct realists] can insist that we perceive complicated dispositional or statistical properties by perceiving their concrete manifestations. These manifestations are concrete properties instantiated by the perceived objects, so it is not surprising that they appear to be simple, intrinsic properties." Yes, indeed we do, and they are, and it is not. But to say this involves accepting the strong division between what belongs to the object as it exists within itself and what appears within the mind. To accept this is to give up naïve or direct realism. What is within the mind is not the same as what is in the object. But if, hypothetically, it were the same, then at best what is in the object would be simple and intrinsic, not dispositional or statistical, contrary to the whole framework of modern natural science. At worst, what is in the object would have the same phenomenal character as what is in the mind, and so materialism would be false. (There is also a side issue about the claim that attributes are *instantiated* by objects. This way of speaking goes more with Plato, or at least Aristotle, than with materialism.)

The point of saying a perceptual impression is "some sort of" awareness is that selective attention must also be taken into account, as William James pointed out long ago. Given the failure of selective attention, the awareness one has with an impression may be weak or only implicit, perhaps below the threshold of effective functioning. But this is not what is at issue with direct versus indirect realism. For selective attention is not about perceiving impressions as though they were themselves objects.

ROBERT FRENCH'S REPLY TO CRITICS

Le Morvan correctly points out that direct realism and naïve realism do not always have the same meaning, and in fact in his contribution has carefully distinguished among a number of different usages of "direct realism." I use the term "direct realism" just to refer to naïve realism as the position that we are immediately aware of the front surfaces of distal objects. While I concede that most modern so-called "direct realists" claim that perception of distal objects occurs in virtue of causal chains linking these objects with the perceivers, I completely fail to see how these linkages make perception be cognitively direct. Perhaps cognition from these chains would constitute indirect evidence for distal features, but I fail to see how this would be direct. In fact I deny that experiences per se are cognitive at all since cognition is a feature of the interpretation of an experience rather than the experience itself, which instead I hold to be spatial.

Le Morvan claims that because I hold that the distinction between the senser and the sensed breaks down I am on the road to some version of idealism or phenomenalism. I wish to stress that this is definitely not the case. In talking about the "senser" and "sensed" here I was just referring to events in phenomenal space. I still hold that numerically distinct distal physical objects of perception exist, but where the sense in which we are said to perceive them is indirect and does not include immediate awareness. Instead I hold that the physical objects of perception here transcend our experience in a sense, which Steven Lehar clearly enunciates in his contribution. I am not as committed as Lehar is to a completely biological explanation of phenomenal experiences, as I prefer to be agnostic on this issue.

Le Morvan also asks for me to clarify what I say concerning reconstructing ordinary perceptual language and suggests that it may be a version of an adverbial account perhaps akin to that of Chisholm (1957). One point here is that objects in phenomenal space are not distal as with Chisholm's account. One example for an active case reconstruction of perceptual language is to say for a region of phenomenal space and time that the region reddens—in the sense of phenomenal red. The copula could also be used here by saying that the region is phenomenally red. I believe that the distinction between phenomenal color and physical color is truly fundamental—for example, phenomenal white is a simple noncomposite shade while as Newton (1754/1952) points out white light is composite and the reflectance properties of so-called "white objects" are also very complex. I also expand on the geometry of phenomenal visual space using spherical polar coordinates in French (1987). It can be admitted that a reconstruction of perceptual language is not very useful for most practical purposes, but the foregoing sketch shows how it can be done.

Schmidt claims that there is a third sense of "direct realism" besides the epistemic and ontological senses, which I distinguish between. I believe that it would be more accurate to say that there are two variants of the ontological sense. One sense (a prescientific or unscientific sense) holds that vision is exocentric working by reaching out to distal objects so that we have immediate contact with their visual properties. Such a sense clearly does not accord with modern science. The second is an endocentric theory and appears to be held by most modern so-called Direct Realists, including Schmidt and Le Morvan (who also raises the issue). Being an endocentric theory this theory is consistent with causal linkages between perceivers and distal objects. It then claims that in some manner (which I am incredibly skeptical of) these distal objects directly present themselves to us in virtue of these linkages. Instead, I maintain that we mistake our experiences of the objects for the front surfaces of the distal objects in these cases.

With respect to what Schmidt says concerning Austin, while Austin does talk about seeing rainbows and mirages, notice that both possess physical explanations even though they are not physical objects. Newton (1704/1952), in Book 1 of his Opticks, for example, explains refraction in terms of the refraction and reflection of water droplets. Also, Austin (1962, p. 25) himself mentions an account of mirages in terms of atmospheric refraction whereby something below the horizon is made to appear above it.

Schmidt also raises issues with respect to my treatment of a phenomenal regress by claiming that it retains a distinction between subjects and events in phenomenal and that there must still be some sort of a relation between the two. My reply is to deny that the subject is distinct from phenomenal space. Instead I hold that the conscious self just is phenomenal space—I make no distinction between them. Admittedly, more needs to be said on matters such as how this ties in with such topics as the nature of the conscious aspects of will and cognition, but I will not address such issues here. This also ties in with Le Morvan's claim that the ordinary language of perception is pretheoretical rather than theory-laden. If he merely means by this that it does not assume the causal theory of perception, I agree. However, by merely including transitive verbs, the ordinary language of perception does assume a distinction between the perceiver and what is perceived. As just noted, I reject this at least for the phenomenal case.

STEVEN LEHAR REPLY TO CRITICS

1. THE PARADIGMATIC DIVIDE

Every one of Huemer's objections to the theory of Indirect Perception can be traced to a profound paradigmatic difference between alternative views of the problem of vision and the entities involved. Fig. 14.1 illustrates the paradigmatic divide with the example of the experience of a view of a table. Fig. 14.1A–C depicts the theory of Indirect Perception, from A: the objective external table as it exists out in the world, through B: the subjective experience of that table viewed from a particular perspective at a particular distance, (with eyes open if the table is within the visual field), to C: (if you think about it) the cognitive inference that *there is a table*. Fig. 14.1D–F depicts the theory of Direct Perception. The key difference is that D represents a superposition of items A and B into a single objective/subjective

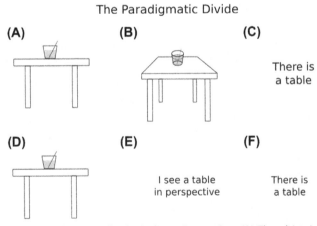

The Paradigmatic Divide

Figure 14.1 The paradigmatic divide. Indirect Perception: (A) The objective table. (B) The subjective experience of the table (sense data). (C) The inference. Direct Perception: (D) The objective/subjective table. (E) Noninferential justification. (F) The inference.

entity that is somehow both the objective external table and also the sub-jective experience of that table. Now Huemer objects vehemently to the notion that the colored surfaces of the table in your experience are part of your experience, even those surfaces are experienced, and are experienced *as surfaces*. To Huemer's view, experience is not an image like item B, experi-ence is a "view" like item E. There is no image in experience but the world itself viewed directly. Except for dreams and hallucinations, they are to be ignored as a special case that has no relevance to this issue.

The problem with merging the objective external table with the table viewed in experience (one a physical object outside your head, the other a spatial experience arguably within it) is that they are easily separable by sim-ply closing one's eyes. The part of the world that blinks out of existence (the entire visual field!) is the internal world of experience causally downstream of your closing eyelids, while the objective external table continues to exist uninterrupted by the closing of your eyelids. How can the one disappear in a blink while the other continues to exist when there is no distinction between them in D? If perception were direct then it would not be blocked by closed eyelids. The very concept of the objective/subjective structure is a direct expression of the Naïve Realist assumption that what you see is what is out there and embodies the paradox of vision in this paradoxical entity that is supposedly objectively real but disappears when you close your eyes. The union of these dissimilar entities into a single concept represents a category error at the most profound level that explains and refutes every objection raised to the existence of sense data.

2. THE CAUSAL ARGUMENT

For example, Huemer objects to the statement that if direct realism is true, then our sensory experiences are spatially located outside our bodies. What Huemer means is that the extended colored surfaces that we observe *in our experience* are not actually part of our experience, they are surfaces out in the world beyond the sensory surface, even though those experienced surfaces go dark when we blink our eyes, and even though dreams and hal-lucinations demonstrate experienced surfaces that are not perceived directly, thus demonstrating conclusively the existence of sense data as independent of objective reality. Tellingly, Huemer does not attack Indirect Perception in the paradigm ABC, but rather he reformulates Indirect Perception to the form DEF, where item E is supposed to represent "sensory experi-ence" but in the absence of an image like that observed in experience. The "experience" E is merely "viewing" the spatial structure D that is perceived directly, out where it lies in the world, not mediated by the sensory pathway. There is no image at all in experience itself, the only "image" present is the objective/subjective world itself D. Except in the case of dreams and hallucinations, in which case the image that is experienced does not actually exist anywhere except in experience. Prominently absent from this explanation of vision is item B, the table as it is experienced subjectively, with spatially extended surfaces with perspective distortion applied, complete with optical illusory effects like the bent stick.

How would the theory of Direct Perception account for a vivid hallucination where an image is experienced that does not exist out in the world? Where is that image located if it is not out in the world? How can we experience an image when no image exists in the world known to science? In fact the reason why Huemer attacks *his* theory DEF instead of the *true* theory of Indirect Perception ABC is because the latter is unassailable when evaluated in fair comparison. Huemer argues as if the concept of sense data was impossible in principle. The existence of dreams and hallucinations conclusively demonstrates the existence of mind-constructed sense data of experience as explicit spatial experiences that are clearly distinct from external objects.

2.1 The Perception Argument

In the Perception Argument Huemer challenges the notion that for me to perceive (e.g.,) a table, it is causally necessary that P1: certain electrochemical processes occur in my brain. Therefore, P2: I cannot perceive an external, physical table; I can only perceive a replica of a table in my head. Huemer claims that P2 does not follow from P1. Well it certainly follows in the case of a video system where certain voltages on particular photosensors represent an image of the world projected on them by the lens, and that therefore the image is located on the photosensor array expressed as a pattern of voltages. The image is not located out in the world beyond the lens because the image is registered on the sensor array behind the lens. What Huemer is arguing is that vision is not representational like a video system, but he fails to provide an alternative explanation for how *visual information enters the mind*, except to say that it is "direct" and self-evidently so, ignoring the obviously representational architecture of the lens, retina, and optic nerve. It does not bother Huemer in the least that nobody has ever constructed a model visual system that can record or register world information except by way of its sensors. What does that even mean? The whole idea of Direct

Perception is a category error at the most profound level, and that is why it is impossible to even conceptualize or demonstrate the principle in an artificial vision mechanism. The principle of Indirect Perception on the other hand is easily demonstrated by every video camera connected to a computer.

Huemer explains "the fact that perception involves events in the brain does not mean that *what we perceive* is something in our brains. What we perceive (the *objects* of our perception) is not to be confused with the process of perceiving, nor with the causal conditions of our perceiving." This statement makes no sense to an Indirect Realist with an ABC view of perception, this argument is only coherent within the DEF paradigm, where item E "views" the external world "directly" in D, where it performs the "process of perceiving" in the absence of any image-like representation in experience. Prominently absent from this explanation is item B, the world of visual experience as it is experienced, complete with perspective distortions already applied.

3. DREAMS, HALLUCINATIONS, AND ILLUSIONS

On the question of dreams and hallucinations Huemer argues that just because hallucinations are illusory does not mean that normal perception is necessarily illusory. Again, what Huemer misses is that dreams and hallucinations are composed of sense data, and thus they demonstrate that sense data *can* and *do* exist, and there would be no purpose for the existence of sense data if they were not involved in perception. Surely the purpose of dreams is not merely for our nocturnal entertainment, they are clear evidence of a constructive or generative process of visual representation also used in normal perception, as confirmed by visual illusions, which contains more explicit spatial information than the retinal stimulus on which it is based. Visual perception is a constructive or generative function, and the world we see around us in visual experience is that virtual world within our brain.

Indeed in visual illusions we often see real and illusory objects combined in the same experience. Are the "real" parts perceived "directly" out in the world where they lie, whereas the illusory parts simply "do not count as real objects" while still being experienced? Again, the only reason Huemer finds his argument persuasive is because he views it through the DEF paradigm where an illusory figure would register in item E, without any kind of image being involved. The fact that we perceive illusory surfaces as extended spatial surfaces demonstrates that illusory experience is image-like in nature and that sense data are real.

Huemer cites the bent stick illusion when a stick is half immersed in water as an example of Direct Perception. Huemer writes "you see the stick (the real, physical stick, for that is the only sticklike thing there is), which *looks* bent but *is* straight. The fact that it looks bent does not mean that it is a stick-replica in your head." Again this explanation is as paradoxical as the phenomenon it seeks to explain. In diagram DEF the "image" of the real stick out there in the world, item D, would be straight, but item E that "views" that stick "directly" sees it as bent. Really? But item E is not an image, just a "view" of item D, so there is no image of the stick as being bent or straight, except in my experience. The bentness neither has objective existence in the world nor in my mind or brain. The paradox of Direct Perception is built right into item D the supposed "subjective/objective" entity that is somehow straight and bent at the same time, without any kind of image involved. All this perplexing paradox simply disappears in paradigm ABC where the real stick is straight in A in a glass that is perfectly circular, while the experience of the stick is bent in B, with an elliptical projection of the circular glass as observed in perspective, and with the square table top appearing as a trapezoid in our experience, while at the same time we perceive the trapezoidal sense data to be actually square because the scale of perceived space shrinks between the near and far sides of the table, and the rear legs are perceived to be shrunken by perspective but to be otherwise objectively the same dimensions as the near legs. Item B provides a full and complete account for the perception of perspective and illusion as it is experienced in our everyday experience. *It is this item that is prominently absent* from the Direct Realist account of visual experience.

4. THE GEOMETRICAL ARGUMENT

On the Geometrical Argument Huemer argues that just because the world appears warped by perspective does not mean that visual space is inside your head, but rather that "visual space does not exist. *Nothing* can have contradictory properties, wherever it may be. Locating an object in a person's head does not enable that object to defy the laws of logic."

Fig. 14.2 shows the paradigmatic diagram for the experience of a railway track. Fig. 14.2A depicts the railway track as it really exists, with tracks parallel and ties equidistant as far as the eye can see. Fig. 14.2B depicts the experience of that same railway track for an observer standing on the track.

The Paradigmatic Divide

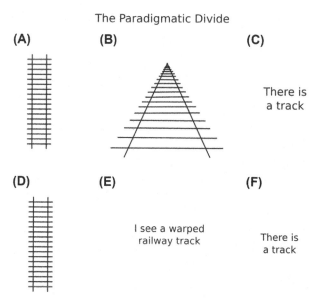

Figure 14.2 The paradigmatic divide. Indirect perception: (A) The objective railway track. (B) The subjective experience of the railway track (sense data). (C) The inference. Direct perception: (D) The objective/subjective track. (E) Noninferential justification. (F) The inference.

Fig. 14.2B depicts a single object with contradictory properties: The tracks are both parallel and equidistant, and yet at the same time they converge to a point. The ties are all the same length and yet they get smaller and smaller at the same time. The "contradictory properties" are built right into the representation itself. This figure, and the visuospatial experience it represents, is an example of a single object that has contradictory properties. Fig. 14.2B is a two-dimensional projection of the actual experience had when standing on railway tracks. In the full three-dimensional case you get a three-dimensional experience wherein the tracks are both parallel, and at the same time they converge to a point, while being perceived to be straight and parallel and equidistant throughout their length. The contradictory property is built right into the geometry of our visual space. If Huemer ignores this aspect of perception, how does he account for the results of the Hallway Experiment? Are the subjects lying? Or can they see something he deliberately ignores? Is Huemer the only one who cannot see perspective distortion when looking down a hallway? Can he really deny that objects in the distance appear smaller in one sense, while at the same time being undiminished in size in another? Is our experience of the world *not* like a museum diorama? With objects in the distance represented at ever smaller scale?

The only way that Huemer could overlook something so obvious is if his observations of his own experience are tainted by his theoretical preconceptions. If you really believe that you are seeing the tracks directly, then they cannot possibly converge, even though they obviously seem to. It is possible to ignore the convergence of perspective: Indeed it is adaptive to do so in real-world interactions, to discount the warp (as Huemer does so well) to more accurately perceive the geometry of the world as it really is through the perspective distortion. But to ignore the obvious convergence of the tracks is to ignore one of the most obvious observational facts of visual experience, a central fact that actually provides vital evidence for how the brain solves the vision problem, if only we are not too blind to see the obvious.

Huemer's argument seems deliberately obtuse in refusing to acknowledge the "contradictory" warp in perspective that is so obvious everyday experience. But to understand how Huemer is thinking one has to think from within the DEF paradigm where the object being observed, the railway track, item D, *is* objectively straight and parallel as far as we can see it, it is only our "view" of that track, item E, that "perceives" the warp somehow, and yet there is no image-like experience involved at all. Prominently absent from this explanation is item B, the track as it appears in our experience, with perspective distortion already applied. Huemer's apparently contradictory explanation stems from the fact that he cannot acknowledge the obvious perspective warp in the railway tracks that the rest of us see since he believes to be perceiving them "directly," so he must assign the warp to item E, the "view" of D, and yet no image is involved in experience, despite the fact that our experience of the railway track is both an experience of an extended structure, and it is a structure with a perspective warp. There is no way that we could be seeing the tracks as warped if we were perceiving them directly.

Huemer argues that "*train tracks receding in the distance sort of appear to get closer together, and sort of appear parallel. But this doesn't show that there is some pair of objects with contradictory properties, whether in your head or elsewhere.*" If they "*sort of appear parallel*" while "*sort of converging*" that is exactly the *duality in size perception* that reveals the world of experience for the internal virtual world that it is. It is not perceived as a "pair of objects," one warped and the other not, it is perceived as a single object that is both warped, and at the same time it is not, as in item B in the diagram, because it exists in a warped space that makes it appear warped when it is objectively not. Huemer's claim that acknowledging this duality in perception commits one to a dualist view of experience is absurd. There is only one space in visual experience, and it is warped.

5. CONCLUSION

The question of the directness (or otherwise) of perception is a classic case of a paradigm debate where the opposing camps argue endlessly at crossed purposes due to different foundational assumptions on the very nature of the problem. But the situation is not symmetrical: The theory of Direct Perception can be placed side by side in fair comparison with Indirect Perception as shown in the paradigmatic diagram. Significantly, Huemer cannot bring himself to characterize Indirect Perception as the paradigm ABC, he must first recharacterize it as paradigm DEF before "defeating" it as implausible because Huemer cannot bring himself to accept the reality of sense data, or the possible existence of extended images in our experience. The item B in the paradigm diagram is, to Huemer's view, a total impossibility, so he will not even discuss paradigm ABC because he claims it to be inconceivable. However, the only evidence Huemer cites for this refusal is that Direct Perception is self-evident. How could it possibly be otherwise? It is a noninferential justification of the obvious: What we see is what is out there. If I see my foot, it is my foot that I see, not an internal replica of my foot, and that in turn demonstrates that perception is direct. This is merely a restatement of the thesis of naïve realism, which is falling victim to the Grand Illusion of conscious experience.

But it is impossible to fairly compare alternative paradigms if you begin from the outset with the initial assumption that your paradigm is right. With that initial assumption you could only ever conclude what you began with in the first place, even if you have to totally redefine the meaning of *experience* and *representation* in the process. But the real-world information that we acquire through the senses is experienced as if from a viewpoint, with perspective distortion already applied, as if viewing through an optical system that presents more distant objects at smaller scale. We experience the color of objects exposed surfaces but neither of their hidden rear surfaces nor of their internal volumes. Why would Direct Perception fail to record the color of hidden rear surfaces of objects or of their internal volumes? Those are also objectively present, why are they not directly perceived? And why would objects in the distance appear smaller (while at the same time appearing undiminished in size) if perception were direct? Is perspective foreshortening not an obviously optical phenomenon?

Huemer provides an able rationalization for naïve realism for those who feel inclined to believe it from the outset. He neither shows why perception *must* be direct nor even how it could *possibly* be direct; he does not even show that perception cannot possibly be indirect; he merely provides a rationalization for those who are already persuaded that naïve realism is not as self-evidently absurd as it actually is. The paradigm diagram compares the two paradigms fairly, revealing the item B, prominently absent from the Direct Realist explanation, and the paradoxical item D, that is experienced to be spatially extended but is not a spatially extended experience, that is experienced to be objectively present but disappears when you blink, that appears to shrink in scale as it recedes into the distance while maintaining its objective size unchanged, and that may not even exist objectively and yet is experienced as a spatial structure. The theory of Direct Perception is not a theory of how vision works, or how we could replicate it in artificial vision systems, it is a theory that embodies all the paradoxes of perception in the model itself, without any hint of a clue as to how an artificial vision system could be devised to enjoy the magical "external" perception that we observe in our everyday experience.

REFERENCES

Austin, J., 1962. Sense and Sensibilia. Oxford University Press, Oxford.
Chisholm, R., 1957. Perceiving: A Philosophical Study. Cornell University Press, Ithaca.
French, R., 1987. The geometry of visual space. Noûs 21, 115–133.
Newton, I., 1704/1952. Opticks. Dover Publications, New York.
Smythies, J., d'Oreye de Lantremange, M., 2016. The nature and function of information compression mechanisms in the brain and in digital television technology. Front. Sys. Neurosci. http://dx.doi.org/10.339/frsys.2016.00040.
Smythies, J., 2017. The role of brain mechanisms in the generation of consciousness. J. Conscious. Stud. 24, 1–2, 254–263.

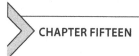

CHAPTER FIFTEEN

Rebuttals by Direct Realists

Robert French

Adjunct Instructor, Philosophy, Oakland Community College, Waterford Township, MI, United States

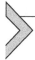

PIERRE LE MORVAN'S RESPONSE TO ROBERT FRENCH'S COMMENTS

Bob is right that I classify indirect realism as a form of perceptual realism. I trust that he would agree that it is insofar as indirect realism takes perception-independent objects to be what we perceive albeit indirectly. It is true that I do not say much about indirect realism (although I am not sure what it inconsistent in what I write about it), but in terms of a division of labor, that is a task I leave to the indirect realist contributors. I mention only paradigmatic indirect realists such as Locke and Descartes but would be happy to acknowledge Russell and Smythies as well.

Bob correctly notes that indirect realism has at least as many variants, and some of these variants (particularly epistemic ones) may even be compatible with some variants of direct realism. This is an important point. Perhaps one of the indirect realist contributors could take on the valuable taxonomic work suggested by Bob's point.

He also makes another very important point concerning a danger that can arise with shifting among different variants of naïve realism. Though a direct realist, I actually agree with him about the danger of such shifting to avoid refutation. Note that I am not *defending* a form of naïve realism here; I think those who call themselves naïve realists need to be a lot clearer about what their position *does and does not* amount to. I do not think there is sufficient clarity about this in the literature, and that is one of my main motivations for the taxonomy I offer in my contribution.

EVA SCHMIDT'S RESPONSES TO DAVID MCGRAW AND ROBERT FRENCH

I would like to thank David Mcgraw and Robert French for their insightful comments on my paper. I will begin by responding to Mcgraw's criticism.

Direct versus Indirect Realism
ISBN 978-0-12-812141-2
https://doi.org/10.1016/B978-0-12-812141-2.00015-5

McGraw addresses my attack on the last escape route for epistemological disjunctivism *sans* metaphysical disjunctivism. His complaint is that—to the contrary of what I claim the epistemological disjunctivist should endorse— when Louis sees the child drowning, what explains his knowledge that the child is drowning is not the fact itself that the child is drowning. It is not *because* of the fact that Louis knows this. For this is "hidden from him" (p. 212). Rather, his knowledge is explained by his perceptual functioning, which makes him aware of the fact that the child is drowning, and thus at best indirectly explained by the fact. I take it that this is an indirect realist claim. According to McGraw, it does not conflict with the idea that the concept of perception is fundamental, so that hallucination is "botched" perception.

Note that my claim was not that, for the epistemological disjunctivist, the perceived fact explains the perceiver's knowledge (though I agree that it does). It is rather that, analogously to the case of action, worldly facts can *justify* and *motivate* beliefs. What makes Louis's action of jumping in the water and saving the child right or what counts in favor of his acting in this way, is that the child is drowning. Further, what moves him to jump in the water is this very fact. In the same vein, this fact makes Louis's belief that the child is drowning right and counts in favor of his so believing. It moves him to adopt this belief. McGraw does not explicitly oppose any of these claims (he talks about explanatory reasons but does not mention justifying/ normative or motivating reasons), but I suspect that he is opposed to them as well. For if worldly facts as explainers of knowledge are hidden from and thus inaccessible to the subject, it stands to reason that they are also hidden from and inaccessible to her as explainers of action and as motivators and justifiers of action and belief.

McGraw's comments do not touch on my argument that the epistemo- logical disjunctivist should allow for worldly facts to be excellent reasons that justify belief. The first point I made with regard to this was that the strong antiskeptical stance that motivates epistemological disjunctivism in the first place is weakened if the view cannot allow that the world itself con- tributes to the excellent justification of our beliefs. I agree with McGraw that a theorist who gives up on this last idea by conceding that the worldly facts are hidden from us can accept that hallucination is a kind of botched perception. But this theorist will thereby also give up on epistemological disjunctivism. However, I tried to raise problems for the *entrenched* episte- mological disjunctivist. I argued that while she can allow that hallucination is perception gone awry while insisting that the mental state of perception provides for our excellent reasons, she thereby gives up on the claim that excellent reasons may be worldly facts to her own grave disadvantage.

The other argument I presented is based on the extremely plausible claim that what counts in favor of, or justifies, certain *actions* are worldly facts, not our experiences of them, and on a parallelism between reasons to act and reasons to believe. This argument does more than spell out what epistemological disjunctivists are committed to. It shows that it is generally desirable to allow that our reasons to believe include worldly facts. How does McGraw's objection affect this argument? As stated above, I agree that the assumption that we are never directly confronted with worldly facts puts pressure on the claim that they can justify or motivate our actions and beliefs. In particular, if we can never be aware that something is the case in our environment, it seems problematic to say that its being the case can motivate us to act or believe a certain way. But if something could never motivate us to perform a certain action or to adopt a certain belief, it is hard to conceive of it as something that counts in favor of this action or belief. For it can not be right that there may be normative reasons for us that we are in principle unable to pick up on.

It thus appears that the indirect realist view briefly sketched by McGraw conflicts with the thesis that worldly facts can be reasons to act and reasons for which we act. Since he gives no argument in his comment for why we should think that reality is hidden from the subject, and since the view that worldly facts can justify and motivate action is extremely plausible, however, this causes trouble for his indirect realist view and strengthens the epistemological disjunctivist proposal.

French suggests that the highest common factor view, into which epistemological disjunctivism is in danger of collapsing, is a version of indirect realism. If this is right, the only available version of direct realism is naïve realism. I think this is a very interesting point. Intentionalists will disagree with French's claim, however—they accept that there are substantial commonalities between perception and hallucination, for they are defined by their shared intentional content. But intentionalists deny that perceivers are in touch with the world only indirectly, for example, by perceiving the intentional content of their experience that then represents their surroundings. Rather, they hold that perception represents the perceiver's environment immediately. That it represents the environment is to say that it has an intentional content; the view is not committed to thinking of the content as interposed between perceiver and environment. Similarly, intentionalists will say that representational vehicles underlie perception; they are needed for the subject to be in touch with her surroundings. But again, this does not commit the view to holding that the subject directly perceives her representations and through them, indirectly, her environment. Maybe intentionalists are mistaken—but French would have to provide an argument why this is so.

Further, French is worried that my argument commits me to propositionalism about perceptual content. I am not so committed (cf. Schmidt, 2015), where I argue that we should ascribe two levels of content to perceptual experience, scenario content, and an external content consisting of worldly states of affairs. I argue for pragmatism about the nature of perceptual content in Schmidt, n.d. Admittedly, in my argument against epistemological disjunctivism *sans* metaphysical disjunctivism, I phrase my references to perceptual content propositionally. My motivation is that, on the one hand, it is convenient to pick out perceptual contents propositionally when talking about perceptual justification. For this manner of speaking suggests a simple account of perceptual justification modeled on belief-to-belief justification, viz. in terms of inferences between believed propositions of the same kind. By contrast, if we think of perception as directed at objects, this opens up a worry about how exactly perception can justify belief if it has this structure, which I wanted to bypass. (I do propose an account of perceptual justification based on the assumption that perception has nonpropositional content in Schmidt, 2015.)

On the other hand, nothing in the argument hinges on how we conceive of perceptual content, as consisting of objects, Fregean propositions, states of affairs, etc. The essentials of my argument are that, given transparency, the excellent, reflectively accessible reason present in the good case exhausts what is subjectively conscious about perception. So there can be no substantial commonalities with hallucination. For this argument, it makes no difference what exactly it is that the excellent reason consists in, for example, whether it is a worldly object or state of affairs (i.e., something nonpropositional). The other horn of the dilemma is that, if we assume that there is a commonality between perception and hallucination with regard to their conscious character, we leave no more room for perception to make an excellent reason reflectively available to the perceiver. Again, the correctness of this point does not hinge on what exactly the excellent reason is, ontologically speaking. It may be an object or a (nonpropositional) state of affairs, for example.

MICHAEL HUEMER'S RESPONSES TO DAVID MCGRAW, ERNEST W. KENT, STEVEN LEHAR, AND ROBERT FRENCH

Michael Huemer

I would like to thank professors David McGraw, Ernie Kent, Steven Lehar, and Robert French for their interesting and valuable comments on my chapter ("The Virtues of Direct Realism," this volume). Here I will make a few brief remarks in reply to their comments.

1. MICHAEL HUEMER'S REPLY TO DAVID MCGRAW

Professor McGraw does not disagree with me, so I have little to say in reply apart from expressing satisfaction at our central agreement. He does, however, go beyond what I said, when he offers a criticism of the "brain-in-a-vat" argument. (This is the argument, given by skeptics, claiming that we cannot know about the external world because we can not prove that we are not brains in vats.) As I understand it, McGraw holds that the skeptic's argument is self-undermining: the brain-in-a-vat argument depends on our knowledge about brains, vats, and so on, but this knowledge is part of what the skeptic himself is rejecting. For instance, the skeptic assumes that *brain activity causes sensory experiences*, but that italicized claim is itself a contingent claim about the external world, so the skeptic denies that we can know it.

Though I share the goal of exposing the errors of external world skeptics, I do not believe that this is among those errors. I do not think the skeptic needs to rely on our knowledge of any contingent facts about brains. Rather, it is enough—so the skeptic would claim—that it is *logically possible* that there be a brain kept alive in a laboratory and stimulated by scientists to produce experiences as of an external world. The skeptic holds that, to know anything about the world around us, we must be able to refute every logically possible alternative (whether or not we have any evidence for that alternative).

The skeptic's argument thus does not rely on any contingent knowledge of the external world. It does not, for example, involve assuming that electrical activity in a brain *in fact* causes sensory experiences in the way that we think it does. The skeptic need not even assume that brains exist. Since it is *logically possible* that brains exist, that brain activity causes sensory experiences, that a computer is stimulating a brain in a vat, and so on, we allegedly need to prove that all this is not happening to us.

So I think the skeptic's error is not one of self-refutation. The skeptic's error is merely that of embracing a false epistemological assumption: the assumption that knowledge requires positive evidence refuting every logically possible alternative.

2. MICHAEL HUEMER'S REPLY TO ERNEST W. KENT

Professor Kent, too, appears not to dispute the substantive views I advanced in my chapter. His point of disagreement appears to be about whether what I have said "has anything to do with Indirect Realism"; he thinks that I am merely attacking "a straw man" and advancing "a trivial truth."

These criticisms are not correct.

First, my use of "direct realism" and "indirect realism," while not the *most common* way in which these terms are used, is far from idiosyncratic. The epistemological issue on which I focused has been widely debated in epistemology for centuries, and it is standard to use the terminology of "direct/naïve realism" and "indirect realism" in describing the opposing positions in the debate; I list several examples in the footnote.[1] So there is no question about whether the issue I addressed has something to do with indirect realism.

Second, the position I criticize—Epistemological Indirect Realism—is by far the dominant view in the history of the subject. Epistemological Indirect Realism was held by such luminaries of epistemology as René Descartes, David Hume, and Bertrand Russell.[2] It continues to be the view of many contemporary epistemologists, such as Richard Fumerton, Laurence BonJour, and Jonathan Vogel.[3] None of these are silly or unimportant thinkers; on the contrary, these are some of the leading figures in the field—including, indeed, some of the leading figures in the entire history of human thought. So a criticism of the view could hardly be an attack on a straw man.

Nor, for the same reasons, could my own view—Epistemological Direct Realism—be described as a trivial thesis. In fairness, Kent did not describe Epistemological Direct Realism itself as trivial. I *think* what he regards as

---

[1] See, e.g., Fumerton (1985, p. 73, 1998, p. 395), Van Cleve (2015, pp. 81–82), Lyons (2017, section 2.1.5), McDermid (2001, pp. 4–5, 7–10), BonJour (2004, pp. 350–351), Huemer (2000, p. 398). For an extended discussion of Thomas Reid's epistemological direct realism, see Van Cleve (2015, ch. 11).

[2] Descartes (1984), Hume (1975), Russell (1997).

[3] Fumerton (1985), BonJour (2004), Vogel (2014).

trivial is the *psychological* thesis that our perceptual beliefs are not based on other beliefs. He goes on to say that this allegedly trivial thesis "proves nothing other than that we all have had essentially the same experiences from which we have learned to have expectations about what we perceive."

That is not correct. It proves something more: when combined with other premises, it supports Epistemological Direct Realism. (These other premises are the Basing Requirement on knowledge, and the premise that we actually have perceptual knowledge.) This is explained in my original chapter, so I will not rehearse the argument here. Kent has not disputed any part of the argument other than the labeling. And the conclusion, again, is something that has been rejected by the great majority of thinkers who have ever addressed the issue. So, whether or not the premise is trivial, the argument as a whole definitely is not.

But the premise is hardly trivial. If we consider only explicit, conscious basing, then it is indeed obvious that perceptual beliefs are not based on other beliefs. That is why I explicitly allowed, in Chapter 10, Section 1, for the possibility of *unconscious inference* and *justificatory dependence without inference*. Recall the example of the belief "I live in the United States": I did not *infer* this from other beliefs, certainly not consciously; nevertheless, it clearly *depends* for its justification on other justified beliefs. Similarly, the sophisticated indirect realist would maintain all our beliefs about the external world depend for their justification on other justified beliefs. It is not obvious on its face that this view cannot be defended. That is why I had to explicitly argue against that possibility in Chapter 10, Section 3.3, rather than merely pointing to the obvious.

Now, why does Kent see no interesting issue here? I suspect the reason is that he has misunderstood the issue I am addressing. To be clear, I am not addressing a psychological issue. I am not asking how perceptual experiences or beliefs are caused. I am not asking a scientific question of any kind. I am asking a *philosophical* question—more particularly, an epistemological one. The question is: how are perceptual beliefs *justified*? Why is it rational, why does it make sense, why *should* one believe in external objects of the kinds we seem to perceive—rather than, say, thinking that there are only the experiences in one's own mind, or that one is a brain in a vat, or that one is receiving ideas directly from the mind of God?

I am not at all convinced that Kent has understood this question. He begins by alluding to "a vast literature on mechanisms of unconscious determinants of perceptual experience." This does not seem on its face to be relevant to the epistemological question.

Kent recognizes that it is not relevant to my question. But I do not think he understands why. Here is his description of the reason: "[Huemer] is only discussing epistemic beliefs and whether they are derived from perceptual experience by inferential or non-inferential means..."

I do not know what Kent means here by "epistemic beliefs." I was discussing perceptual beliefs—for example, the belief that there is a table in front of me. I would not have called that an epistemic belief. It is not, for example, a belief about knowledge, nor is it any particularly special sort of belief. It is just an ordinary belief about the physical world.

Be that as it may, I am not only discussing whether these beliefs "are derived from perceptual experience by inferential or non-inferential means." My central question is, again, what *justifies* perceptual beliefs, not what *causes* perceptual beliefs.

Now, this point may have been obscured to some degree because what causes perceptual beliefs is in fact *relevant* to what justifies them. The fact that the two questions are closely related, however, should not lead one to confuse them with one another. I used premises about how perceptual beliefs come about, but that does not mean that my *thesis* is a thesis about how perceptual beliefs come about; I used those premises to *support* a *normative epistemological conclusion*, namely, that perceptual beliefs have a kind of foundational justification, explained by the principle of phenomenal conservatism. I find no clear evidence that Kent has understood this.

3. MICHAEL HUEMER'S REPLY TO STEVEN LEHAR

Professor Lehar appears, if anything, to understand my views even less than Kent does. Nearly everything Lehar says about my views is false. I believe the version of "direct realism" that he ascribes to me is a straw man: I do not hold that collection of views, and I doubt that anyone ever has.

To be specific: I do not hold that an experience of a foot *is* a foot, nor do I deny that there are experiences of feet. I do not posit any "objective/subjective" entities that are both mental and physical at the same time. I do not deny that appearances can be deceiving. I do not deny that there are causal preconditions on perception, both in the external world and in our bodies; thus, I do not think that the mere existence of an external object is sufficient for us to perceive it. All these views that I do not hold strike me as ridiculous and in no way suggested by anything I have said. Finally, I do not say that direct realism is self-evident. I do not think that would be a *ridiculous* view, but I did not assert that view in my chapter.

I also do not have a confused view of indirect realism; I do not, for example, think that indirect realists deny the existence of sense data or of mental images. I do not think they hold that we only have abstract beliefs about the external world instead of experiences of it.

As an aside, Lehar thinks that my view of perception is represented by items D-E-F in his diagram, but that I *think* indirect realists actually believe the D-E-F story. If that were so, why would I think I disagreed with the indirect realists? If the view that I ascribe to them is really my own view, then would not I just praise the indirect realists for getting things right? Be that as it may, I do not believe the D-E-F picture, nor did I ascribe it to indirect realists or anyone else.

What led Lehar astray? At one point, I referred to the indirect realist's view that perceptual beliefs depend for their justification on "propositions about mind-dependent phenomena." Lehar appears to have interpreted this to mean that I think indirect realists deny the existence of actual experiences and that I think sense data are supposed to be just abstract beliefs without any qualia. He protests that this view removes the imagistic nature of sense data.

Rest assured, I was never so intellectually incompetent as that. I never doubted that sense data are supposed to be imagistic. Nevertheless, [I am having experience E] is a proposition, *no matter what E is like.* E can be as imagistic as you like, with as many sensory qualia as you like, or whatever other properties you want to ascribe to it. The fact that you are having *that* experience is still a "proposition," that is, a thing that is either true or false. This point has nothing whatever to do with the issue between direct and indirect realism and nothing to do with my arguments for direct realism in the chapter.

Now, what is my actual position? And what am I ascribing to the indirect realists? My view cannot be understood by looking at the name "direct realism" and then importing whatever associations the reader initially has with those words. Rather, what I mean by "direct realism" and "indirect realism," in my chapter, is simply *and only* what I stipulated that the terms mean in that chapter. Here is what I stipulated (this time, I include the adjective "Epistemological" for extra clarity):

Epistemological Direct Realism: Perception provides noninferential justification for external world propositions.

Epistemological Indirect Realism: Perception provides only inferential justification for external world propositions.

I further explained that, for a belief to count as having inferential justification, it is enough that its justification *depend on* other justified beliefs, even if the thinker did not actually infer it from those other beliefs; see Chapter 10,

Section 1 in my original chapter. Now, most of what Lehar says in his comment has nothing to do with this issue. So I will pass over those parts.

I gave two central arguments for Epistemological Direct Realism: the argument from the Basing Problem and the Symmetry Argument. Lehar says nothing about the Basing Problem. So the first of my two main arguments stands thus far undisputed.

Lehar offers a response to the Symmetry Argument: he says that the difference between sensory appearances and other kinds of appearances is that sensory appearances are imagistic, while other appearances are more intellectual (presumably, he is thinking only of intuitions and reasoning, not of memory or introspection).

But this reply by Lehar simply forgets what the issue was. The issue was not whether there is *any difference at all* between sensory appearances and nonsensory appearances. The issue was whether there is a reason why nonsensory appearances can justifiedly be presumed correct, whereas sensory appearances cannot be trusted until there is positive evidence of their reliability. *That* was the asymmetry to be justified. And what Lehar says here simply does not address that. Lehar gives us no hint of why we are epistemically permitted to presume that intuitions (or memories, or introspective judgments, or logical inferences) are correct until proven otherwise but not entitled to presume that sensory appearances are veridical until proven otherwise. Simply saying "sensory appearances contain images" does not answer that.

Thus, the Symmetry Argument has not in fact been addressed. This being the case, we should not posit an epistemological asymmetry between sensory and nonsensory appearances; we should treat all appearances the same. As explained in Chapter 10, Section 4.1, this means we should be Epistemological Direct Realists.

Lehar does offer one objection specifically to Epistemological Direct Realism. Here it is:

> But sensory appearances can be deceiving, most clearly in the case of dreams and hallucinations, so they can hardly serve as an ultimate source of justification for anything except for the existence of the experience itself, as it is experienced to be.

The argument appears to be this, in brief:
1. Sensory appearances are fallible.
2. Therefore, sensory appearances do not provide noninferential justification.

But I addressed this already in Chapter 10, Section 4.2. To review, I pointed out (1) that the argument is simply a non sequitur, and (2) that premise 1 could be applied equally well to any other sort of appearance, and thus the argument would force one into global skepticism.

Lastly, there is one other argument of Lehar's that I would like to address, even though it does not appear relevant to Epistemological Direct or Indirect Realism. This is the argument that if you close your eyes, you stop seeing objects; therefore, perception cannot be direct. (Lehar actually says that "part of the world [...] blinks out of existence," but this is obviously false. You merely stop seeing part of the world.)

This argument is not only irrelevant to Epistemological Direct Realism but it is also, to the best of my knowledge, irrelevant to any form of direct realism that anyone has ever advanced. For no form of direct realism that anyone has ever held claims that there are *no causal conditions* on perception. When you close your eyes, you stop perceiving the physical world. That does not imply that when your eyes are open you do not perceive the physical world, nor does it imply that you perceive (or otherwise have awareness of) some nonphysical things instead.

Now, Lehar thinks that direct realists have trouble explaining *why* we stop perceiving objects when we close our eyes. But direct realists have no trouble explaining this: the reason is that closing your eyelids prevents light from reaching your retina. There is nothing about direct realism (whether it be Epistemological or Ontological) that remotely conflicts with that obvious explanation. The process of reflected light reaching your retina, electrical impulses traveling down the optic nerve to your visual cortex, and the electrochemical activity that then occurs in your brain—all of that is part of how you perceive objects. And it just obviously does not follow from any of that that (as Lehar claims) you never perceive a physical object. That whole process *is what it is* to perceive a physical object.

4. MICHAEL HUEMER'S REPLY TO ROBERT FRENCH

Robert French ascribes to me the view that "experiences are external world propositions and thus [...] conceptual." This view would contain two confusions, one of them a very gross category error. Fortunately, I am not so confused as that.

Propositions are things that can be true or false; can be asserted, denied, believed, doubted; and can be possible, probable, implausible, and so on. When a person has a belief, there is something *that* the person believes to be the case; that thing is called "a proposition." For example, when you believe that squirrels are furry, your belief is directed at the proposition [squirrels are furry]. Notice that the proposition is not a mental state. The thing *that* you believe is not the belief; there is no such thing as a belief that is about nothing but itself. It also is not a word, series of words, concept, collection of concepts, or experience; all those ideas would be gross category errors. The belief, in this example, is about *squirrels* and the furriness thereof; it is not about words, concepts, beliefs, experiences, or anything else like that. So I would never say that an experience *is* a proposition.

I do, however, say that experiences may represent propositions as being the case. If you see a red tomato, it will typically look red to you. So your experience represents the tomato to be red. That the tomato is red is something that is either true or false, i.e., "a proposition." This is not some arcane, controversial thesis that I came up with because of my weird views; this is simply a direct consequence of the trivial fact that we perceive things as having characteristics.

I also do not say that propositions "are conceptual." That is another serious confusion.

At the same time, I confess that I have not understood French's view either. He says, for example, that "illusions are constructed in phenomenal visual space." I do not know what "phenomenal space" is, nor what it means to "construct" something in it. I rather suspect that "phenomenal space" is a term with no referent.

French, like Lehar, suggests that ordinary people commonly mistake an *experience* or *appearance* for a physical object or the surface of a physical object. This strikes me as a bizarre sort of error for a person to make since it would be confusing two utterly different kinds of thing, like confusing a dog with a color. An experience is a kind of *mental state or event*. It is not even in the same broad metaphysical category as a physical object. Physical objects have sizes and shapes and masses; they occupy the environment around us; you can sit on them, kick them, eat them, and so on. None of these things are true of *experiences*. So it seems unlikely that we are constantly confusing experiences with physical objects. Here, it seems to me, is a more plausible hypothesis: we are normally aware of the physical objects around us, rather than our experiences. We do not, in the normal course of events, perceive experiences at all, let alone attribute to them properties that they can not possibly have.

Now to turn to my arguments for Epistemological Direct Realism, one of my central arguments was the Basing Argument: only direct realism can account for ordinary people's *knowledge* of the external world because only direct realism grants us a justification for those beliefs that plausibly matches why we actually hold them.

In response, French holds that "it is possible for an indirect realist to rationally reconstruct senses of 'knowledge' in non-illusory contexts that work for at least most practical purposes." I believe the suggestion is that the Epistemological Indirect Realist can offer a definition of "know" that allows us to count as "knowing" things about the external world, where that definition comes *close enough* to capturing the ordinary sense of "know" in English. French concedes that we cannot (on an indirect realist view) attain *certainty* about external world propositions, but he suggests that we can attain sufficient reliability. (He also mentions "pragmatic accounts" but gives no details.)

This, however, does not address the main thrust of my argument. True, my argument concerned the inability of indirect realists to account for our knowledge. But this problem had nothing to do with certainty; I did not, for example, say that the indirect realist's problem is inability to give us certainty in our beliefs about the external world. Rather, the problem stems from the Basing Requirement for knowledge: a person counts as knowing something only if they believe it, they have an adequate source of justification for it, *and their belief is based on that justification.* In other words, roughly speaking, you have to believe something for a good reason. This is a pretty weak requirement for knowledge; notice that it is nowhere near as strong as a requirement of absolute certainty. But the Epistemological Indirect Realist cannot satisfy it; he denies that the actual basis of most people's perceptual beliefs constitutes a legitimate justification.

So the idea of rationally reconstructing a sense of "knowledge" would only help if we were to devise a definition of "knowledge" wherein you do not even need to believe P for a good reason to count as knowing P. Of course, one can grant oneself the right to say one "knows" whatever one wants, as long as one is willing to stretch the meaning of the word "know" far enough. I can only say that, in this case, this strikes me as stretching too far from the ordinary usage of "know" in English to be interesting. Direct realism has the advantage that it does not require any such stretch for us to lay claim to knowledge of the world around us.

FRED ADAMS, GARY FULLER, & MURRAY CLARKE REPLY TO ROBERT FRENCH AND ERNEST W. KENT

We are happy to address the concerns brought by Robert French and Ernie Kent to our defense of direct perception. We will first reply to French and then give our reply to Kent.

French's main concern seems to be our remark that as direct realists we are defending that perception is a two-placed relation and that we see indirect perception as committed to a three-place relation. French denies that his "representational realism" involves a three-placed relation and claims his view too involves a two-placed relation—since, he too denies that there is an object in between the perceiving subject's experience and the distal object of perception.

French maintains that a subject's experiences "are constituted by events in a private phenomenal space." We are not sure what a phenomenal space is, if it is not a representational space. And if it is a representational space, then it is either produced by a set of neural events in the perceptual areas of the brain or somewhere else in the causal chain of perception. If it is neither of these, then we really do not know what it is. However, if it is a neural representational space in the perceptual cortex and if, qua representation, it generates a representational space (French's qualitative space), then we are not sure how his view differs from ours. There exists two relata: the experience and the distal object experienced. That is our view. If this is French's view too, then kumbaya! We can all rejoice. However, he claims NOT to be a direct realist but a representational realist. So he needs something to differentiate his view from ours. And if it is not the insertion of another relatum in the perceptual chain, then, frankly, we have no idea what it is that distinguishes his view from ours—direct perception.

He also says something quite puzzling: "It is not so much that reconstructing perceptual language solves the regress as that it created it in the first place by forcing a distinction between perceivers and what is perceived, by using transitive verbs." Now if there is a collapse between perceiver and perceived then French is not only a direct realist but also an idealist. Perhaps he is a nonphysicalist about the mind such that both the mind and the world perceived are mental stuff. Then the perceiver and perceived might be one, but short of that, we have no idea what he is saying. In our example of Matt's experience of the feel of the keyboard, the experiential feel is the perceiving, the keyboard is the perceived. How could these possibly "collapse?" Matt's experience consists of things going on in his head. What he experiences (the keyboard) is not in his head. We simply have no idea how these could collapse for a physicalist. And if they do not collapse and French is still not a direct realist, then despite his protests to the contrary, there simply MUST be a third thing somewhere in his account.

Indeed, we think French's own words prove our point: He says:

In contrast to the version of direct realism of Adams et al., I hold that neural events in the brain – neural correlates of consciousness - produce a reconstruction of certain features of the distal object in a private phenomenal space. I then hold that in ordinary life, using the common sense attitude of naïve realism, we then take (or better mistake) the private phenomenal spatial experience for the distal object. As I point out in my paper this works for most, but not all (e.g., cases of compelling illusions), practical purposes.

The produced "reconstruction" is the third thing. There is the external physical object (relatum #1). This object is *the what* that we say is perceived. For French, in addition there is then the reconstruction of the distal object. This for French is *the what* that is perceived (relatum # 2). And there is *the taking* (relatum #3).

As for French's remarks about "qualia" in the phenomenological tradition, we are happy to take his word for it but that does not change our minds or our usage of the term. He quite well understands our usage and knows that we are following the usage of Dretske (1993, 1995) and Tye (1995, 2009).

Lastly, we maintain that you directly see the image in the mirror and indirectly see the object reflected. Similarly for live TV. You see the image on the screen and only indirectly the objects at which the cameras are pointed. What is more, we deny that we are mistaking objects in phenomenal space for anything. French's phenomenal objects are objects, which have *representational reality only* (as Descartes knew, long ago). They have *intentional existence* (or inexistence) as Brentano knew. But the objects of perception have genuine physical existence as everyone knows. Hallucinated snakes have no physical existence. Real snakes do. We keep them separate. When we see real snakes, the representations may be qualitatively similar, but we do not mistake the representation for the real thing. Representations of snakes have no venom.

Turning to Kent, "a central criticism of his seems to be that our account cannot handle the 'full nature' of qualitative experiences" (Kent, 2017, p. 2). Kent asks: "I want to know whether the information in the neural state of affairs does or does not contain all of the information necessary for the phenomenal experience."

The answer is yes. It does in so far as the information allows the neural state to represent the distal object and its properties and in that it establishes the qualitative feel of the experience.

To his "Why do we need something else?" we say that we do not need something beyond the perceptual experience of the perceiving subject. The phenomenal content comes from the objective external properties being represented by the neural state. To Zach, the stop light looks red because it is red and Zach's perceptual neural events represent the redness. What it means to represent is explained in more depth and detail in Tye (1995, 2009) and Dretske (1995, 1993) than we can provide here.

Something more? Ah yes, there is the business of "recruitment" the selection by the brain for events that carry information about the properties of the distal objects. This intrabrain selection is the key to understanding the representationalist's view of qualia. It is too much in this short reply to go into depth about this view, which is explained in detail by the references cited above. Still, we can say a bit about it in the following paragraphs. It is important to stress at the outset that there is nothing mysterious or "mystifying" about this view. It is quite physicalistic and naturalistic and biological.

Kent's worry about phenomenal content is handled by appeal to the idea of recruitment. Rob's experience has the content as of a snake because it was recruited to have the function of carrying information about snakes. In normal circumstances, Rob's snakelike experience does carry that information. Rob could still be in such a perceptual state, however, even if he is having a hallucination or an illusory experience and "even if the perceptual state can no longer perform its function" (Dretske, 1995, p. 75).

Appeal to normal circumstances helps to deal with a related concern of Kent's. Our account of direct perception helped ourselves to Dretske's notion of the object that is *primarily represented* by perceptual experience. For us, in the normal case when Matt tactilely experiences the *F* key what is directly represented is the distal key and not the signals being sent along the circuits of the receptors. Because the information about the *F* key may be carried by way of multiple pathways the tactile experience does carry information about the signals. The *F* key is the first object in the causal chain about which the tactile experience carries *nonequivocal information*.

We agree that veridical, illusory, and hallucinatory experiences, e.g., as of a bent stick or of a snake, may all be qualitatively similar (see our p. 37). Kent's worry seems to be this. Our account, he thinks, explains phenomenal content in terms of the information carried by the experiential state. But the information carried by such qualitatively similar states is different. Rob's alcohol-induced hallucinatory experience carries no information about actual snakes! So, our account fails to fully explain the nature of qualitative states. But this is not true. Nonveridical experiences of snakes do not carry information about any actual snakes. At most they carry information about the property of being a snake but not an actual snake because none is actually perceived.

About the bent stick, we do not understand Kent's objection. Light bends in a medium of water. Light sets up the correlation between stick and experience. Thus the experience of the stick looks bent—period! There is nothing mystical here either.

We do need to say a bit more here about our account of qualitative state in terms of representational state. In the bent stick illusion case, the "qualitative" representation is different from the representation in the case where the stick is in a glass with no water; we can handle the difference in terms, not of what the actual object is but in terms of the differences between the medium of light moving through air and moving through water!

Kent argues that our account of direct perception is wrong by appeal to the jiggling eyeball example. In this case the world, e.g., your parked car, which is actually stationary, seems to move. On the primary representation account of direct perception in this case what is directly perceived is the moving retinal image (moving because the eyeball is moving). The moving retinal image is the first object in the chain about which the experience carries information. But surely the visual experience is about a moving car.

Our reply here is as follows. We need to distinguish between what the content of the experience is from what the experience is directly about. Of course, on our Dretskian recruitment account the content of the moving eyeball experience is *as of a moving car*, but what the experience is directly about is in this abnormal case is still the nonmoving world. But the experience is mediated by a moving image on the retina of the jiggling eyeball.

We did express the above point early in our article, when we said that "[i]t may be possible (perhaps when one's arm 'falls asleep' or under the influence of certain kinds of drugs – LSD) to experience the nerve firings and give them primary representation, but this is not the case when Matt is in normal states and using his computer" (p. 6). In this case of Matt's tactile experiences under these abnormal conditions, we would say that the content of Matt's experience was as of the *F* key, but the direct object of the experiences was the nerve firings.

When you jiggle your eyeball, the WORLD does not move. Your eye moves and its movement affects the correlation between perceptual state and world. Thus, it appears to move because the medium of perception moves, via the moving eyeball. Still nothing mystical here.

Kent gives his own story about how an internal model would explain things when the eye jiggles, but on our view no internal model perceived is needed. That is why ours is a two-placed relational model, not a three-placed, as is his.

On our view the "out-there-ness" when we look at the coffee cup is due to both the perception of the cup and the space around it and perhaps of the proprioceptive feedback of reaching for it. In any case, it is due to the direct perception of the cup in space. There is nothing more to it than that. Everything else is overintellectualizing the (what French terms "ontic") perceptual process.

As for perception of color, there is nothing yellow in the brain. So from whence comes the experience of the yellow daffodil? Why, from the yellow daffodil of course!

We have given our reasons for denying that we perceive Kent's internal models. That requires a three-placed relational view of perception. We prefer the two-placed relational view. We will let science and history decide which view is correct. All we can do is give the reasons for our preference. After that, everyone gets to pay their money and take their chances.

Fred Adams (University of Delaware)

Gary Fuller (Central Michigan University)

Murray Clarke (Concordia University)

REFERENCES

Adams, F., Fuller, G., Clarke, M., 2017. Seeing Things: Defending Direct Perception. (This volume, nn-nn).
BonJour, L., 2004. In search of direct realism. Philos. Phenomenol. Res. 69, 349–367.
Descartes, R., 1984. Meditations on first philosophy. In: Cottingham, J., Stoothoff, R., Murdoch, D. (Eds.), The Philosophical Writings of Descartes, vol. 2. Cambridge University Press, Cambridge.
Dretske, F., 1993. Conscious experience. Mind 102, 263–283.
Dretske, F., 1995. Naturalizing the Mind. MIT/Bradford, Cambridge, M.A.
French, R., 2017. Reply to Adams et al. (This volume, nn-nn).
Fumerton, R., 1985. Metaphysical and Epistemological Problems of Perception. University of Nebraska Press, Lincoln, Nebr.
Fumerton, R., 1998. Externalism and epistemological direct realism. Monist 81, 393–406.
Huemer, M., 2000. Direct realism and the brain-in-a-vat argument. Philos. Phenomenol. Res. 61, 397–413.
Hume, D., 1975. An enquiry concerning human understanding. In: Selby-Bigge, L.A. (Ed.), Enquiries Concerning Human Understanding and Concerning the Principles of Morals. Clarendon, Oxford.
Kent, 2017. Reply to Adams et al. (This volume, nn-nn).
Lyons, J., 2017. Epistemological problems of perception. In: Zalta, E.N. (Ed.), Stanford Encyclopedia of Philosophy, Spring 2017 ed. https://plato.stanford.edu/archives/spr2017/entries/perception-episprob/.
McDermid, D.J., 2001. What is direct perceptual knowledge? A fivefold confusion. Grazer Philos. Stud. 62, 1–16.
Russell, B., 1997. The Problems of Philosophy. Oxford University Press, New York.
Schmidt, E., 2015. Modest Nonconceptualism: Epistemology, Phenomenology, and Content. Studies in Brain and Mind Series, vol. 8. Springer, Cham.
Schmidt, E. (n.d.). "Can We Do Without Content Pragmatism?" (manuscript).
Tye, M., 1995. Ten Problems of Consciousness. MIT Press, Cambridge, M.A.
Tye, M., 2009. Consciousness Revisited. MIT/Bradford, Cambridge, M.A.
Van Cleve, J., 2015. Problems from Reid. Oxford University Press, Oxford.
Vogel, J., 2014. The refutation of skepticism. In: Steup, M., Turri, J., Sosa, E. (Eds.), Contemporary Debates in Epistemology, second ed. Wiley-Blackwell, Malden, Mass, pp. 108–120.

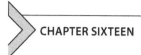

CHAPTER SIXTEEN

Postscript

Robert French[1], John Smythies[2]

[1]Adjunct Instructor, Philosophy, Oakland Community College, Waterford Township, MI, United States; [2]The Center for Brain and Cognition, University of California San Diego, La Jolla, CA, United States

We wish to thank the contributors on both sides of the debate for keeping their remarks nonpersonal and sticking to the issues with respect to what admittedly are highly contentious issues about which participants on both sides have strong opinions.

The dispute between direct and indirect realists may seem to be just a battle over best explanations where admittedly each side has to buy into at least one seemingly incredible claim—which is that causal links with distal objects make these objects "present themselves" to us in the case of the direct realists, and the claim that phenomenal events can be accounted for either in terms of neurobiology or some form of dualism in the case of the indirect realists. We believe that it would be unfortunate just to leave matters here. We also believe that it is a mistake for either side to just declare victory at this point.

The issues discussed in this anthology are truly fundamental. It is also clearly the case that the respective positions of at least metaphysical direct and metaphysical indirect realism are mutually incompatible—e.g., on the topic of whether conscious perception consists of a "presentation" of nonmental distal objects (either in virtue of causal connections with these objects or by a prescientific "reaching out" to these objects), or, instead, is a phenomenon involving "reconstruction" of aspects of physical distal objects by specific representative mechanisms. In view of this incompatibility we suggest that more needs to be done to clarify these matters.

No matter how you slice it the truth is extraordinary. On the indirect realist side this involves either postulating that neural states possess a phenomenal aspect to them (which goes beyond traditional neurobiology) or that there is a connection with phenomenal space in some other manner (as suggested, for example, by new forms of substance dualism). On the direct realist side this involves the ability to "reach out" to distal physical objects in the past, whether in virtue of causal linkages with those objects or in some other manner not at present explained. Likewise direct realists need to

Direct versus Indirect Realism
ISBN 978-0-12-812141-2
https://doi.org/10.1016/B978-0-12-812141-2.00016-7

explain in detail how we see only what the brain computes is most probably "out there" rather than what is actually "out there"—in particular how the visual data compression mechanisms recently discovered in neuroscience operate in their system of explanation.

We believe that the philosophy of mind (aided by constructive input from the neurosciences) needs to focus on investigating these ideas and not just accepting the dystonia between them. Otherwise there is the danger of the philosophy of mind becoming irrelevant and slowly going out of existence, at least as a separate discipline apart from neuroscience.

On the converse side we believe that neuroscience needs to examine its own metaphysical assumptions, particularly concerning the nature of space, time, matter, and causality, very carefully. These assumptions contain positions that seem "obviously true" yet, on further examination, critical doubts as to their verity can legitimately be raised. One example of these is the idea held tenaciously by almost all neuroscientists that particular neural events are identical to particular phenomenal events—which may be challenged if we apply Leibniz's law of the identity of indiscernibles. Another is the widespread belief among visual neuroscientists that the stimulus field (containing the physical objects that we see "out there") is the same entity as the visual field (what we experience in consciousness). This entails holding two mutually incompatible theories (direct and indirect realism) at one and the same time. This leads to the absurd position that the input to a computation can be identical with its output. Neuroscientists tend to support indirect realism in their laboratories and direct realism as soon as they get home.

INDEX

Printed in the United States
By Bookmasters